Hidden Fears, Helpful Memories:
Aftermath of the 1983 Bombing of the
United States Embassy in Beirut

A Thesis
submitted in partial fulfillment of the requirements for the
degree of
Master of Arts in Liberal Studies

By

Anne Dammarell, B.A.

School for Summer and Continuing Education
Georgetown University
Washington, D.C.
November, 1994

Copyright © 2024 by Anne Dammarell

All rights reserved. No part of this publication may be reproduced, distributed, or transmitted in any form or by any means, including photocopying, recording, or other electronic or mechanical methods, without the prior written permission of the copyright owner and the publisher, except in the case of brief quotations embodied in critical reviews and certain other noncommercial uses permitted by copyright law. For permission requests, write to the publisher, addressed "Attention: Permissions Coordinator," at the address below.

CITIOFBOOKS, INC.
3736 Eubank NE Suite A1
Albuquerque, NM 87111-3579
www.citiofbooks.com
Hotline: 1 (877) 389-2759
Fax: 1 (505) 930-7244

Ordering Information:

Quantity sales. Special discounts are available on quantity purchases by corporations, associations, and others. For details, contact the publisher at the address above.

Printed in the United States of America.

ISBN-13:	Softcover	979-8-89391-373-6
	eBook	979-8-89391-374-3

Library of Congress Control Number: 2024920635

HIDDEN FEARS
HELPFUL MEMORIES

Aftermath of the 1983 Bombing of the
United States Embassy in Beirut

ANNE DAMMARELL

Table of Contents

ABSTRACT I
PREFACE III
ACKNOWLEDGEMENT VII
DEDICATION IX
LIST OF ABBREVIATIONSLIST OF ABBREVIATIONS XI
CHAPTER 1 : INTRODUCTION 1
The Bombing and its Context 1
Thesis and Methodology 3
CHAPTER 2 : POST-TRAUMATIC STRESS DISORDER 7
Diagnostic and Statistical Manuals 8
Post-Traumatic Stress Disorder Symptoms 8
Critical Incident Stress Debriefing 9
CHAPTER 3 : PERSONAL RECOLLECTIONS 12
Memory of Bombing 12
Personal Reaction to the Bombing 16
CHAPTER 4 : FOREIGN SERVICE OFFICERS' RECOLLECTIONS 24
A.   INTERVIEWS WITH FSOs 24
FSOs' Immediate Reaction to Bombing 25
Impact of Bombing on Foreign Service Officers 32
Views on Why the Embassy was Bombed 37
Preparation for Danger Posts 40
Follow-up Support After the Bombing 43
B.   QUESTIONNAIRE COMPLETED BY FSOs 49
Preparation for Beirut Assignment 50
Reaction to Bombing 50
Follow-up Activities After the Bombing 51
C.   SUMMARY OF FINDINGS 53
CHAPTER 5 : INSTITUTIONAL PROCEDURES AND REACTIONS ... 56
State Department Procedures in 1983 56
Inman Report in 1985 57

State Department Procedures in 1994 58
CHAPTER 6 : CONCLUSIONS AND RECOMMENDATIONS 62
Conclusions 62
Recommendations 64
APPENDICES 66
A LIST OF INTERVIEWEES 67
B. INTERVIEW - OPEN-ENDED QUESTIONS (11/93) 68
C FOREIGN SERVICE OFFICERS WHO WERE SENT
      QUESTIONNAIRE 70
D. QUESTIONNAIRE 71
E. SURVIVING AMERICAN EMPLOYEES IN BEIRUT47 81
F. LEBANESE STAFF KNOWN TO HAVE DIED 84
G. MISSING STAFF PRESUMED TO BE DEAD 85
H. INJURED STAFF 86
I. LIST OF THOSE INTERVIEWED 87
J. INTERVIEWS 88
ENDNOTES 170
BIBLIOGRAPHY 175

Abstract

The first U.S. Embassy destroyed by political terrorists exploded in Beirut on April 18, 1983. Seventeen Americans died. Sixty-seven survived. Unfortunately, little has been written about that event.

This paper discusses the type of preparation the Foreign Service Officers (FSOs) had for serving in a danger post and how they reacted to the bombing and processed the event.

To collect this information a select number of FSOs were interviewed and sent an anonymous questionnaire. Department of State officials responsible for the educational and medical programs were also interviewed.

The FSOs who were in Lebanon in 1983 unknowingly experienced post-traumatic stress disorder symptoms similar to those faced by war veterans and victims of trauma. Although the Department of State attempted to address the needs of the survivors, it did not provide sufficient training and follow-up support to allow them to recognize, acknowledge, and fully process the trauma.

Many FSOs had not been prepared for working in a war zone and, when caught up in the bombing, they continued work, "business as usual," without fully acknowledging the traumatic effect the bombing had on their lives. As a result, they may have delayed the process of healing the psychological wounds caused by the explosion. FSOs did not pressure the Department to provide additional psychological support because many either saw no need for it, or did not value the concept of psychiatry and/or the competency of some of the psychiatrists working within the Department.

The vast majority of FSOs experienced—and some still do today—a series of post-traumatic stress reactions; however, only one FSO described symptoms which may indicate a full-blown post-traumatic stress disorder. The FSOs were not educated in the psychological ramifications of trauma. Although most FSOs instinctively worked through their emotional reactions by talking to colleagues and family, all may not have processed fully their reactions to the bombing. Some may not have acknowledged the need to recognize and process the trauma of the bombing.

The Department of State does not officially acknowledge that violence has a long- term effect on those involved, even if only indirectly involved. The predominant Foreign Service culture has yet to rid itself of the outdated attitude that any attention to mental health betrays a weakness. The notion that using the services of educators and counselors as a form of preventive medicine and a way of educating oneself on normal human development has not caught hold.

Preface

Terrorism has become the preferred-perhaps only-way that the weak and impotent nations can conduct war against the powerful, the rulers of the world. In recent years, terrorists, with quick-strike flexibility and reliance upon theatrical symbolism, have zeroed in on the diplomatic community. For the United States, they have escalated their ante from targeting ambassadors, to the capturing of the an embassy full of ready-made hostages in Iran in 1979, and finally to the double bombing of our embassy in Lebanon in 1983 and 1984.

Throughout this process a subtle yet deep structural transformation of how Foreign Service Officers operate has taken place. Since terrorists view diplomats as combat personnel, embassy security has increased and embassy staff find it increasingly difficult to be as open and as relational as previously. Embassy as fortress is no mere metaphor. In some countries, it is reality. Unlike members of the armed forces, however, Foreign Service Officers working inside the embassies receive little support or training to prepare them for battle and its aftermath.

I was in the first bombing of our embassy in Beirut in the early afternoon of April 18, 1983 and one of only two survivors in the cafeteria. Although seriously wounded, years slipped by before I accepted the reality of my injuries, because I did not want to believe that my physical capacity had been limited and that my life had changed. Yet my life had changed profoundly: I had felt the pain and isolation of a near-death episode and had gained insight into the brevity and joy of life. At age forty-five, I had confronted my own mortality. Ten years later, I am still plumbing the meaning of that experience.

The bombing was dramatic and, perhaps, the most significant event of my life. Because I had been directly involved in this international act of terrorism, I decided to write about it for my master's thesis. When I started my preliminary literature research on the political ramifications of the bombing for my paper, I discovered that very little had been written on the bombing. Surprisingly, I found no books and only a few articles on an event that altered not only our foreign policy but also the way in which our embassies and staff are protected. Why was there so little data? I felt like someone had died but no one had bothered to put up a tombstone.

While I was working in the Georgetown University library, the Marines were preparing for the tenth anniversary of the bombing of their seaside barracks in Beirut. The two hundred and forty-one men killed on October 23, 1983 would be honored at Arlington Cemetery and at Camp Lejeune. Book titles about this Marine tragedy kept popping up on the computer screen as I tried to track the Embassy explosion. I began thinking about my colleagues who had died. I also thought about my colleagues who had lived. What were their thoughts on the tenth anniversary of the bombing? How did the explosion affect their lives? How did they handle the injury and death that had surrounded them? Could their experience be of help to the men and women living in danger posts today?

Al Alexander,[1] on temporary duty assignment from the Department of Commerce, and Consular Officer Philo Dibble[2] gave accounts of the day. Written shortly after the bombing, the articles give little insight into what people were thinking. The stories of the Foreign Service Officers (FSOs) in Lebanon have not yet been recorded.

Stephen E. Auldridge, a Vietnam veteran and Foreign Service Officer writing about the Embassy bombing, said

> The paradox between Nam and Beirut is all there: an unseen enemy, whom we cannot conquer, a Stateside public which does not fully understand, and the seemingly [sic] thanklessness of it all for the price we pay serving overseas.
>
> I remember the feeling of losing "brothers" in Vietnam and crying a frustrated, angry cry. I remember going home and feeling frustrated and angry...It's been 10 years since I remember that cry for lost "brothers," but on April 19 it happened again. The same cry, the same frustration and anger...And now I must again feel

that pain, sharing a grief with all other Foreign Service people over the loss of our own...I knew I wasn't grieving alone...[3]

I changed the focus of my thesis. I decided not to do a political analysis of the bombing, but would write on the reactions of FSOs who were the hidden victims of that ordeal. My personal experience of the bombing differed from those of whom I interviewed, in that my injuries required a series of operations and prolonged physical therapy. Although several colleagues had been hurt, none required hospitalization. Another difference was that I left the "group" four days after the bombing and did not have the post- bombing experience of being in Beirut with colleagues who shared a trauma.

Chapter One describes the bombing and the political context within which the event took place. It also examines the thesis, research procedures and methodology used.

Chapter Two is about Post-Traumatic Stress Disorder.

Chapter Three contains my personal experience of the bombing, which I wrote to help me (and the reader) understand my reactions to the event.

Chapter Four gives the reactions of the FSOs to the bombing and how it affected their lives. (A more detailed account of each person is in the Appendix.)

Chapter Five has the Department of State reactions and procedures to the bombing.

Chapter Six has the conclusions and recommendations.

Acknowledgement

The professors at Georgetown University, whether experts in the psychology of trauma or past teachers, were gracious and generous in discussing my thesis with me. None was more helpful and supportive than my mentor, John Ruedy, whose knowledge of and love for the Middle East has enriched the thinking of many Georgetown students.

By interviewing the Foreign Service Officers who survived the Beirut bombing, I hope to acknowledge all Foreign Service Officers and especially the seventeen Americans killed in 1983:

    Robert C. Ames

    Thomas Blacka

    Phyliss N. Faraci

    Terry Gilden

    Kenneth E. Haas

    Deborah Hixon

    Frank J. Johnston

    James F. Lewis

    Monique Lewis

    Staff Sergeant Ben H. Maxwell

    William McIntyre

    Corporal Robert V. McMaugh

    Staff Sergeant Mark E. Salazar

    William Sheil

    Janet Lee Stevens, journalist

    Sergeant First Class Richard Twine

    Albert N. Votaw

Dedication

To Leona Fisher, Ph.D, of Georgetown University, who encouraged her students in "Theory and Methods of Interdisciplinary Research" to pursue with passion their topics of research and to question why certain subjects and people are not recorded in the annals of history.

LIST OF ABBREVIATIONS

AID	Agency for International Development
AUB	American University of Beirut
AUH	American University of Beirut Hospital
CLO	Community Liaison Office
CISD	Critical Incident Stress Debriefing
DCM	Deputy Chief of Mission
DS	Diplomatic Security, State Department
DSM	Diagnostic Statistical Manual of Mental Disorders
FS	Foreign Service Institute
FSO	Foreign Service Officer
GSO	General Services Office(r)
NEA	Near East and Asia Bureau, State Department
NSC	National Security Counsel
PAO	Public Affairs Office(r)
PLO	Palestinian Liberation Organization
PNG	Persona non grata
PTSD	Post-Traumatic Stress Disorder
R&R	Rest and Recuperation
RPG	Rocket Propelled Grenade
RSO	Regional Security Office(r)
SOS	Security Overseas Seminar
TDY	Temporary Duty
UNICEF	United Nations International Children's Emergency Fund, now known as the U.N. Children's Fund

UNWRA   United Nations Relief and Works Agency for Palestine Refugees in the Near East
USIS   United States Information Service

CHAPTER 1

INTRODUCTION

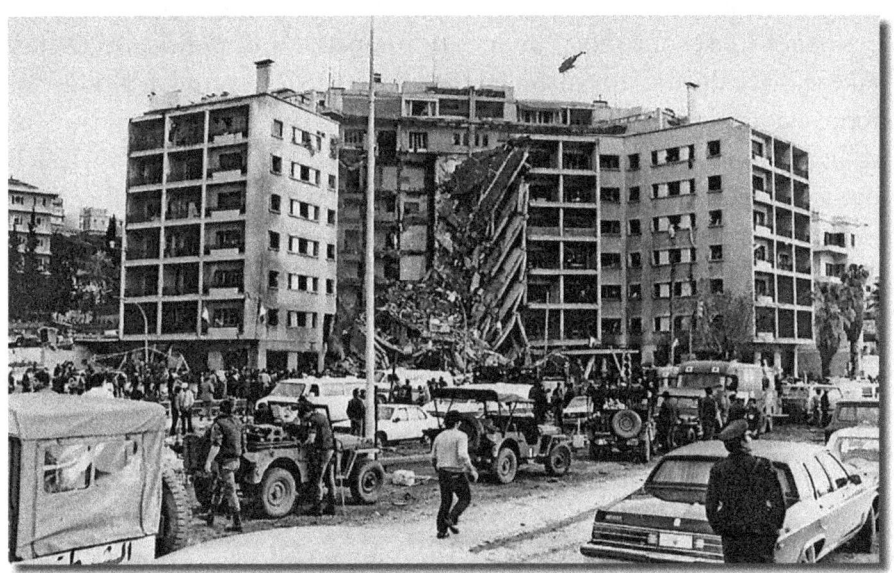

The Bombing and its Context

On April 18, 1983, at 1:05 p.m. a truck, weighted down with over 2000 pounds of TNT[4], drove into the front door of the U.S. Embassy in Beirut and exploded. The core of the building pancaked to the ground: the first American Embassy had been destroyed by political terrorists. Seventeen Americans and thirty-three Lebanese employees were killed. An estimated sixteen visa applicants and passers-by also died. A message had been sent to Washington: leave Lebanon.

At the time the U.S. Embassy was bombed, fighting had been going on in Lebanon for eight years. The Civil War began in 1975 when both the Palestinians and the Lebanese Muslims, in conjunction with the Druzes, challenged the authority of the Christian- controlled government. The political and social structure set in place in 1943, when Lebanon essentially ended the French Mandate, began to crumble. Alliances were made among the various confessional groups of Muslims, Christians, and Druze, depending on the political issue at hand. The fighting was international in nature, as well as domestic. Neighboring Syria, Jordan, and Israel had a vested interest in Lebanon's borders, water supply, and status as host to the Palestinians and the Palestinian Liberation Organization (PLO).

Lebanon also became the "stage" for other Middle Eastern countries to act out their support or disapproval of political activities taking place during this turbulent period. In 1979 Ayatollah Khomeini returned to Iran giving leadership for the rise and exportation of militant Islam. That same year the U.S. supported Egyptian-Israeli peace treaty was signed and the U.S. Foreign Service Officers in Teheran began their four-hundred and forty-four days of captivity. In 1980 Iraq invaded Iran. The next year Egyptian President Anwar Sadat was assassinated by militant Muslims and Israel annexed Syria's Golan Heights. During this time, the U.S. was steadfast in its support of Israel and its opposition to the Soviet Union.

In the late 1970s, under the Begin administration, Israel began an accelerated program of moving Jewish settlers into the West Bank and Gaza, with the goal of consolidating Israeli hold and destroying the PLO's authority. Ariel Sharon, the main architect of this policy, also designed the Israeli invasion of Lebanon in June, 1982, with the same goal of uprooting the PLO, then based in West Beirut and southern Lebanon. Consolidating his troops on the outskirts of Beirut, Sharon had hoped to coordinate plans for the Maronite forces to enter the Palestinian strongholds in West Beirut. However, his advisers rejected this proposal, believing that the Maronites were militarily incapable.[5] In its attempt to broker a peace agreement between Israel and Lebanon, the U.S. began to press for the immediate withdrawal of the PLO. Israel began to shell Beirut continuously which resulted in heavy losses for Lebanon. Alexander Haig, the U.S. Secretary of State at that time, "approved these tactics, viewing Israeli actions as a means of pressuring Arafat to agree to leave."[6] Haig's support of the Israeli plan led to his resignation in late June, and President Reagan's special envoy, Philip Habib, went to Lebanon to negotiate the withdrawal of the PLO. By late August, a multinational peacekeeping force of Americans, French and Italians arrived in Beirut to coordinate the departure of the PLO and to ensure the safety of their families who remained. Once the PLO was evacuated, the force left.

The following month, on September 14, president-elect Bashir Gemayel was assassinated, presumably by the Syrians, because of Gemayel's willingness to recognize Israel. But this has not been established beyond a reasonable doubt. Two days later, Israeli troops entered Beirut and guarded the Palestinian refugee camp of Sabra-Shatila, while the Phalangist (Christian) fighters[7] spent three days massacring hundreds of Palestinian civilians. The multinational forces, including the U.S. Marines, returned after the killings.

In spite of Sabra-Shatila, the U.S. Congress demonstrated its support of Israel by increasing foreign aid to that country. In an attempt to resolve the Lebanese situation, the new Secretary of State, George Shultz, began to negotiate a Lebanese-Israeli agreement in which Israel would agree to withdrawal from Lebanon, on the condition that Syria would do the same. But many Lebanese saw America as firmly on the side of Israel even while U.S. forces on the ground were ostensibly neutral. At this point, the U.S. Embassy was bombed.

Hussein al-Musawi was linked to the bombing.[8] He was the radical activist who broke away from the Shiite militia AMAL to establish the Islamic AMAL in Baalbek in the Bekaa, home to the Iranian backed Hizballah. The general consensus seems to be that Iran and Syria supported Musawi. As noted by Robert Fisk in his book on Lebanon, *Pity the Nation*, the Beirut bureau of Agence France Presse got a call from someone just ten minutes after the explosion claiming that the operation was part of the Iranian revolution's campaign against the imperialist presence.[9] Syria, by this time, was well entrenched in Lebanon political affairs and little could take place without her approval.

Thesis and Methodology

In fulfilling the requirements for a master's degree from the Liberal Studies Program at Georgetown University, I took the opportunity to talk to my friends: not "old shoe" friends from childhood days, but acquaintances dating back only a decade, those Foreign

Service Officers (FSOs) who had been in Lebanon ten years earlier. I wanted to listen to their stories about the bombing of the Beirut Embassy. Stories are powerful, entertaining and transforming. Writer Nancy J. Napier believes that stories about personal trauma are gifts to your future self:

> Every time you go inside and make connections with parts of yourself you set things in motion that develop naturally in a healing way over time. You give yourself permission to create healing whenever you retell a traumatic event.[10]

One goal of this study was to discern the thoughts and experiences of the Beirut FSOs, with the aim of converting their ordeal into something beneficial to the officers presently serving overseas in danger posts.

I am neither psychologist nor psychiatrist. I did not attempt to diagnose any of the interviewees, but simply scanned their responses for post-traumatic stress reactions. As an aside, however, I myself, as a retired Foreign Service Officer, would welcome professional research on the impact of terrorism on the lives of Foreign Service Officers. Unfortunately, a 1983 topic is still relevant today since international terrorism continues to plague Americans abroad.

The thesis of this research is that the Foreign Service Officers who were in Beirut when the American Embassy was bombed unknowingly experienced post-traumatic stress disorder (PTSD) symptoms, similar to those faced by war veterans and victims of other trauma. Although the Department of State addressed the needs of the FSOs, it did not provide sufficient training and follow-up support to allow them to acknowledge and to recognize, acknowledge, and process the trauma.

Research questions included: What impact did the bombing of the U.S. Embassy in Beirut have upon the lives of the Foreign Service Officers in Lebanon? What suggestions do FSOs have for preparing colleagues for danger posts? What did the State Department do to help FSOs deal with the stress of the bombing? What training was given to prepare FSOs for possible terrorist attacks? What type of training does the Department offer today? What reasons do FSOs give for the bombing?

In addition to interviewing the Foreign Service Officers, I talked with State Department officials in the Medical Division, Diplomatic Security, the Family Liaison Office, Employee Consultation Service, and psychologists and several psychiatrists specializing in post-traumatic stress disorder.

I also attended the two-day Security Overseas Seminar (SOS) conducted by the Foreign Service Institute Overseas Briefing Center, and watched the videotapes on stress management and the grieving process produced by Marilyn Holmes of the State Department.

To limit the parameters of my thesis, I restricted my sample to those working for the State Department, the United States Information Service, and the Agency for International Development. My hope was to talk to all those FSOs who were in the United States when I began my research in the winter of 1993. I did not interview members of the Habib[11] peace mission, the Department of Commerce, the Central Intelligence Agency, the Marine security guards, the Defense Attaché's office, military training team and, with the exception of one woman, those on temporary duty.[12] None of the spouses of the FSOs were interviewed, unless they themselves were officers.

By word of mouth and with the assistance of the staff at the Foreign Service Lounge in the State Department, I spoke with fourteen of the eighteen people in the States. The remaining four, although registered with the Foreign Service Lounge, had not authorized the release of their addresses. The staff sent them my letters of inquiry. One responded saying he would answer a questionnaire but did not wish to be interviewed. I did not hear from the other three. I met with those who lived in the Washington, D.C., area and telephoned those who lived out of town.

Interviews, which were taped, ranged from one to three hours. The interviews were transcribed. Some were fifty pages, double-spaced.

For the sake of clarity and brevity, I edited the interviews. These abbreviated interviews do not necessarily follow the order of the conversation. For the most part, they are arranged in the following order: the bombing, personal reaction, opinion as to why the Embassy was bombed, and suggestions for preparing Foreign Service Officers for possible terrorist activity. Each account, reduced to approximately ten pages, double-spaced, is in the appendix. A copy of the questions I posed during the open-ended interviews is attached in the appendix.

One of the members of the Defense Attaché's mission learned of my research and contacted me. Although his data were not incorporated in the study, his interview is also included in the appendix.

Even though I was not able to speak with the Foreign Service Officers posted overseas, they, as well as their colleagues in the States, were sent an anonymous questionnaire. A compilation of the responses is in the appendix.

I collected information from various sources: documentation, archival records, open- ended interviews, an anonymous questionnaire and a State Department training program. The bulk of the documentation came from books, magazines, newspaper articles, and videos dealing with the 1983 bombing and with post-traumatic stress reactions. The archival records were limited to private letters and personal journals concerned with the bombing. I interviewed Foreign Service Officers, government officials, psychologists, and psychiatrists. The interviews with the Foreign Service Officers were taped with their permission. None of the standard questionnaires designed for studies by mental health specialists working in the field of post-traumatic stress disorder was used. They did not meet the needs of this study. I developed a questionnaire especially for the Foreign Service Officers serving in Beirut when the Embassy was bombed.

In conclusion, I limited my study to a set number of FSOs and did not extend it to spouses and children of the FSOs interviewed, Lebanese employees, the military, and other FSOs who were in Beirut at the time. Nor does the study include information on how international and American organizations such as the United Nations, the Red Cross, the Federal Bureau of Investigation, the police, and firefighters are currently addressing the phenomenon known as post-traumatic stress disorder. Little is known about how FSOs and their families process trauma. No baseline data on the kinds and duration of stress which they encounter exist. I hope this thesis will generate interest in and encourage serious research in this topic.

CHAPTER 2

POST-TRAUMATIC STRESS DISORDER

Post-traumatic stress disorder (PTSD) is not a disease, but a reaction to severe trauma. The term "PTSD" is relatively new. The American Psychological Association first codified the syndrome in their 1980 publication, *Diagnostic and Statistical Manual of Mental Disorders (DSM)*. The name came into being to describe the symptoms of Vietnam veterans returning to the United States during the mid-1970s. Initially, the syndrome was referred to as "delayed stress reaction,"[13] because veterans often did not report their problems immediately following combat trauma but only after several months or years. PTSD is widespread among Vietnam veterans. Writer Shirley Dicks, who has interviewed Vietnam veterans with PTSD, estimates that during the course of their lives, more than half will have the disorder.[14] Veterans are often unaware of the syndrome and its origin.[15] The condition, known earlier as "shell shock," was applied to military who had difficulty adjusting to civilian life following the two World Wars and the Korean war. Medical records also document PTSD dating back to the Civil War. PTSD is not limited to the military but affects civilians as well, especially those involved in disasters, police work, and emergency medical, fire and hospital services.

The theory behind PTSD is that, as long as the impact of a trauma is unresolved and its significance is not integrated into the life of the person who experienced the trauma, the affective response to the stress is incomplete and continues to control behavior.[16] Stress is characterized by a wide range of cognitive, physical, emotional and behavioral signs.

PTSD challenges the belief held by some psychoanalysts that the cause of pathology lies only in childhood trauma. This is one reason why the psychiatric community was reluctant to establish a special category for PTSD.[17] Those who suffer PTSD need not have had any previous childhood trauma, repressed or acknowledged. The current *DSM* states that the disorder can develop in people without any preexisting psychopathological conditions, particularly if the stress is extreme.[18] For example, a study of the people in Killeen, Texas, who witnessed the 1991 mass murder of men and women in a cafeteria, showed that most of the survivors with PTSD had no history of prior psychiatric disorders.[19]

Diagnostic and Statistical Manuals

According to the 1987 *Diagnostic and Statistical Manual of Mental Disorders (Third Edition-Revised) (DSM-III-R)*,[20] the main feature of PTSD is the development of characteristic symptoms following a "psychologically distressing event that is outside the range of usual human experience."[21] The nature of the event would be distressing to nearly anyone and is usually a cause for intense fear, terror, and helplessness. The most common traumas include the following situations: threats to one's life or physical integrity, or to the lives of family members or close friends; the destruction of homes or communities; or the witnessing of someone being killed or injured. Types of trauma that trigger PTSD include natural disasters such as earthquakes, accidental disasters such as train wrecks, and deliberately caused disasters such as terrorist bombings. The man-made disasters frequently result in the most severe and lasting disorders. Symptoms of PTSD often begin immediately after the trauma but can be delayed for months or years. When this is the case, avoidance symptoms have generally been present. A diagnosis is currently not made if the symptoms last less than one month.

The American Psychiatric Association is presently revising the *DSM-III-R*. The 1994 edition will include a new diagnosis of Acute Stress Disorder, which is similar to PTSD. The major difference is that Acute Stress Disorder is resolved within four weeks after the traumatic event. When symptoms persist beyond a month, PTSD may be present.

Post-Traumatic Stress Disorder Symptoms

A diagnosis of PTSD is made when a person persistently experiences a combination of at least six symptoms which fall into categories of re-experiencing the event and avoiding the event.

Re-experiencing the trauma takes various forms. If at least one of the following is persistently re-experienced, PTSD may be indicated: unwanted recollection of the event, distressing dreams, flashbacks—a phenomenon in which the person actually believes that she or he is reliving the event (not just viewing it again, as a movie)—and psychological distress at exposure to events that symbolize the trauma.

Avoidance of stimuli associated with the trauma, or the numbing of general responsiveness, in at least three of the following ways also may indicate PTSD: efforts to avoid thoughts or feelings about the trauma, efforts to avoid activities or situations that remind one of the trauma, inability to recall an important aspect of the trauma, diminished interest in significant activities, feeling of detachment toward others, restricted range of affect, or a sense of a foreshortened future.

The presence of any two of the following symptoms of arousal (stress) would complete the syndrome known as PTSD: difficulty falling or staying asleep, irritability or outburst of anger, difficulty concentrating, hypervigilance, anxiety, exaggerated startled response, or physiologic reaction to events that symbolize the trauma.

Critical Incident Stress Debriefing

Jeffrey T. Mitchell, Clinical Associate Professor of Emergency Health Services at the University of Maryland, works with emergency service personnel, such as firefighters and police, whose routine jobs involve life and death scenarios. Mitchell is concerned with critical incident stress management.

Mitchell speaks of three types of victims of a traumatic incident: the primary, those directly affected; the secondary, those who observe the incident or who become part of the rescue crew; and the tertiary, those who are indirectly involved, such as family members. Denial, he says, is perhaps the most commonly used initial defense mechanism. Victims often

> resist special assistance programs because they fear they would be perceived by colleagues and the public as mentally weak and unstable if they admitted to feelings of anxiety. They are quick to suppress their emotions and present a calm facade.[22]

In 1983, Mitchell developed a method of debriefing emergency service personnel. Following a traumatic event, victims are debriefed to assist them in recovering from the impact of the critical incident and to reduce stress symptoms. The debriefing is primarily a group discussion about the event, focusing on how the people involved have managed and how they are presently coping. Known as critical incident stress debriefing (CISD), the confidential session is ideally conducted within twenty-four to seventy-two hours after the trauma and lasts about two or three hours.[23] CISD is conducted by a specially trained team which includes mental health professionals and peer support personnel.

Mitchell divides the formal CISD into seven phases:

1. Introductory remarks
2. Fact phase (what happened)
3. Thought phase (ideas people had)
4. Reaction phase (the worst part of the experience)
5. Symptom phase (types of symptoms experienced)
6. Teaching phase (information on and suggestions for reducing impact of stress)
7. Reentry (questions and answers, closure)

CISD is neither psychotherapy nor a substitute for psychotherapy, but rather a group discussion based upon the principles of education and crisis intervention.[24] Some members of a CISD group may very well seek counseling at a later date, should they discern the need to do so. Mitchell stresses that once post-traumatic stress disorder develops, only an experienced mental health professional should be consulted.

CISD is used routinely by many emergency service personnel in this country, as well as in Australia, Canada, Germany, Great Britain, New Zealand, and Norway.[25] Mitchell notes that some emergency workers resist admitting to any psychological problems to maintain a macho image.[26] Nevertheless, Mitchell claims that CISD hastens the rate of "normal recovery, in normal people, who are having normal reactions to abnormal events."[27]

Dr. Bonnie Green, Director of Trauma Studies at Georgetown University Hospital, noted that reactions to natural disasters last about a year, but reactions to person-caused events can last for years. She advocates a series of debriefings for all who have been involved in a traumatic incident. People can then monitor themselves, she says, to determine what next steps to take. Each one processes trauma differently. In the words of Marilyn Holmes, a writer-producer of training videos for the Department of State,

> Processing trauma, handling trauma, is not like cooking a cake. There are no absolutes. We are all different. The ingredients may be the same, but the measurements are different.[28]

Although debriefings are currently popular and considered helpful, little empirical evidence to support the success of CISD has yet been gathered. However, a study of Australian emergency service, welfare, and hospital personnel showed that CISD did reduce stress symptoms mainly by talking, especially talking with those who experienced the same incident.[29]

Chapter 3

PERSONAL RECOLLECTIONS

Memory of Bombing

Not a jot of chef salad remained. My plate was a circle of white when the bomb exploded.

Five days later, I looked up at Nurse Lake—a black man from Cincinnati—and asked for a chef salad. From the American Embassy cafeteria in Beirut to the intensive care unit of the Army Hospital in Wiesbaden, that salad stalked me. Weeks later, what did I pencil across the oblong menu each morning as I practiced block letters at Georgetown Hospital? Yep. Chef salad.

That happened ten years ago, and I am still plumbing my psyche for the meaning of chef salad. I am not surprised that food is part of my story. But chef salad? Why not tabouli? or baklava? Or any of those succulent dishes that made Lebanese meals last hours.

Bob Pearson, an Agency for International Development colleague, and I were having lunch in the Embassy on April 18, 1983. In those days, people talked about peace breaking out as if eight years of civil war could blossom into a bunch of forsythia. The Israeli invasion, the PLO departure, and the arrival of the multinational forces had disassembled the city's mafioso-like protection system. Beirut, a sea of anarchy filled with islands of disciplined troops, was on Bob's mind. Pushing his cup of *maasboot*, a "just- right-not-too-sweet" coffee, across the table, he said, "Anne, it's not just here, it's all over. This is either the end of the world or the Second Coming."

BOOM.

Mighty loud thunderclap, I thought. Oddly, I didn't hear Bob's expected laugh.

Encircled in blackness, I felt waves of electricity push through my body. I was inside heat—a heat hotter than the oven that blasted my face when I checked a Thanksgiving turkey at age nine. My brain decoded lightning. The Embassy's been hit by lightning. I've been electrocuted! Those damn contractors cheated. They put the fusebox in the cafeteria and a live wire hit my head. I had logically mapped out a scenario. Conscious, I leaned over to tell Bob that I was dead. Only I had no body.

No light. No sound. No one to touch. No God. Nothing. I was alone. A pain, non-physical, deep and psychological, permeated me. No, this is not what they told me death was like. I can't take this for eternity. Anger started to fill my isolation. That was when I flew out—along with the side of building—across the Embassy garden. My body twisted eastward and landed fifteen feet away from where I had just finished my diet chef salad. I don't remember the flight.

I snapped awake within seconds. Alert. A slab of concrete covered my face and body. Claustrophobic, I panicked. I've got to get out of here, I thought, as the adrenaline kicked in. Calm down, Anne. Just last month, a man was found after being buried alive for a week. You just have to push that wall away. My self-lecture helped me focus. Inexplicably, my arms had the force of Jello and were three chapters behind my thoughts. I willed them into sync with my brain. The "slab" broke into bits of brick as I picked open a window. A sweet blue sky assured me of an air supply. All was silent. Then a bird chirp. Calmly, I removed the rubble from my face and chest. I even paused to play with the tacky mixture of blood and dirt, and I watched a glob separate into peaks as I pulled my right index finger away from my thumb. I stared at dust-laden grass camouflaged with debris. A few stubby blades stood up green and clean and out of place. Just like in the movies, I mused. My jaw ached. My right eye was sealed, yet I could see through streaks of blood. Anne, your lid must be cut open. I relaxed.

My chest was numb, weighted down. I looked at the mass of purple-red blood congealed on my left side. Has my heart been ripped from its cavity? My God, I don't have long to live. Hurry, Anne, touch it to see if it's still beating. But I couldn't swing my right arm around to feel my chest. Anne, be reasonable. You would have bled to death if that clump were your heart. Must be a punctured lung. That's all. You can live with one lung, Anne, but you've got to get out of this little grave of yours. Push yourself up onto the ledge, just like in a swimming pool.

Only then I noticed that my legs were pinned down by an air-conditioner. "Bob," I croaked. He is young and strong and can pull that thing away and free me, I thought. I called out twice again. No answer. He's dead. Got to do this by yourself.

Calling Bob's name seem to improve my hearing. The moaning of two men forced me to turn my head to the right. A backdrop of orange activated the scene. Something was still going on. The elongated curtains of fire looked strong and straight like a dramatic prop for an opera. The brick corners of the cafeteria held up empty space. I wondered why the corners stayed up. Why didn't they fall down with everything else? I wasn't afraid, just curious. The fire was far away. Better see what else is happening, Anne. I turned my head to the left.

An even breeze was pushing a long picket-fence of flames towards my head. Imprisoned in my shell, I knew my hair would catch fire first. Fear cleared my head of observations. I had only moments to accept death. I heard the groans of dying men and the song of birds. I pleaded with the heavy black cylinder of smoke circling up from behind me to come quickly and suffocate me. But it began to dissipate, smudging the soft blue sky.

Not fair. Joan of Arc got to suffocate before she burned. So this is the end of my life. Father will have to endure it. How untimely for a child to die before a parent. I felt an achy sadness. No big regrets. Just a sense of not taking advantage of everyday things. I regretted my small and petty meannesses. Remorse for sins of omissions, we Catholics might say.

Again, a strong wish to live pushed me to call for help. I mustered a feeble noise. Blaming myself for not knowing how to say help in Arabic, I hit upon using French. I rehearsed. Say, *secours*. *Secours*. Say *secours*, Anne. I panted in air to energize myself for one loud shout. Opening my mouth, I cried out, "Help." No. No. No. French, not English. I resumed the struggle. I worked to get my breath, my brain, and my mouth to cooperate. "Help," again jumped out before my body slumped in disappointment.

"*Yallah, yallah, yallah* (Let's go)." I heard a strong voice off to my left. Four young Lebanese came running towards me. One, in army fatigues, skidded to a stop and stared at me. He planted the butt of his rifle next to his left foot and assumed the at-ease pose. His gaze went beyond me. He saw what I was too low to see: a room full of dead people.

Drop that damn rifle. You fool. The rifle is in the way. Drop it. Pick me up. Voiceless, I tried to will him into action. The men didn't seem to know what to do. Then one took charge. He told the others to stamp out the flames and leaned over and pulled at my left shoulder. The pain was sharp and pervasive. "Air conditioner," I whimpered. He shouted something. The soldier dropped his rifle and helped the other two men remove the metal from my legs. They brushed off more of the chunks of wall and pulled me out. My body became rigid. The pain stopped. Their arms were like wooden slats of an old-fashioned bed. I rested freely, knowing I was safe. They ran with me past the piles of stone, and I saw for the first time how broken the garden was. I shut my eyes to make the time go faster. Suddenly, one of them tripped and I felt my head falling backward. Anne, get ready. Your head is going to hit the ground. It will hurt, but that's all right. You are safe now, I told myself. My hair gently brushed the ground. The leader started shouting again. This time he was yelling at an ambulance pulling away. They swung me inside like a sack of cement. Someone lay to my right, but I could no longer turn my head. I looked forward. A Lebanese woman crouched over me, saying, "You're going to be all right." I wanted to tell her that my left lung was punctured. I was desperate to make her understand. She leaned forward to read my lips. When she repeated, "You're going to be all right," I knew she couldn't hear me. So I concentrated on the route the ambulance was taking to the American University Hospital. We were going the long way around. Why didn't we take the short cut? Finally, I realized we were pulling up to the hospital grounds. I had been there many times during the past couple of years talking to the staff about emergency supplies and food distributions for the people of West Beirut. Even before we came to a complete stop, the doors were flung open and I was pulled onto a stretcher, rushed inside the lobby and put on a gurney. I saw doctors and nurses racing in. Some had on white coats, others suits. A nurse took my blood pressure.

I was surrounded by people crying, yelling, moaning. A man had taken charge and was telling the nurse what to do with all of us. I was moved to the side. Then down another bit. And then further down, away from the man with the stern voice. He's doing triage. Am I beyond repair? Had my heart been ripped out after all?

Personal Reaction to the Bombing

Two people in the cafeteria survived the blast: my colleague, Bob Pearson, and I. Bob had a possible hairline fracture of his spine, head and face lacerations, a partially detached retina, and shrapnel embedded in his head. I sustained nineteen broken bones, lacerations, and chunks of glass in my neck.

On April 22, I was medevaced to the Army hospital in Wiesbaden, Germany, where my sister Elizabeth Simon joined me. On the third day, I asked to see a psychiatrist to find out why I was not grieving for my dead colleagues. I also wanted advice on what to expect. Working in Beirut during its civil war had been stressful. The bombing only compounded the strain. As I recall, the psychiatrist asked if I had had a religious upbringing. Upon learning that I was a Roman Catholic, he said that I would deal with the ramifications of the bombing after my bones had healed. At the time I did not question him, but I thought his words useless and impractical. My sister Elizabeth noted in her journal that on April 25, 1983, Dr. Baskaran, the psychiatrist, had said it was necessary to be spiritually stable to be emotionally whole, and that all the stages of trauma would come once the body was ready. When I was secure, bodily and emotionally, feelings of anger, grief, and loss would surface. At present, he indicated, I was in the "ego stage" and would focus on mending my bones.

Five days later, Elizabeth and I flew to Washington, D.C., on a military transport plane. I checked into Georgetown Hospital for surgery and months of physical therapy.

I had to relearn how to move my body, to walk, to write, and to focus on the printed word. Walking was difficult, since I could not figure out how to make my feet go. It was not just a question of a fractured pelvis and a broken foot. Tears would blur my vision as I formed my name in spidery block letters across the hospital menu. I felt that I had been flung back into kindergarten and all the intervening years had been wasted. Reading was impossible, as I discovered when the Agency for International Development sent me a form to complete. I stared at the black print and little squares but could not decipher the puzzle. Propped up in bed, I cried until someone came into my room and took the paper away.

Being totally incapable of caring for myself was hard to accept and, quite unconsciously, I evoked childhood stories and adages to aid in my recovery. I had been programmed in the nursery. The chant of Toot, the Little Engine that Could, "I know I can, I know I can,"[30] became my mantra. The cliché of getting back on the horse that throws you motivated me to return overseas as soon as possible.

Both my arms had been broken in several places, but only one required corrective surgery. Following the operation, I once again worried about not mourning those who had died. I wanted a quick fix, not an in-depth analysis of my imperfections. At the time, I thought all psychiatric counseling meant long-term Freudian analysis. Hoping to minimize ethnic, religious, and sexual differences, I asked to see an Irish Catholic woman psychiatrist. Dr. Margaret Clancy came to the hospital and said that she had a box of Kleenex in her office whenever I wanted to schedule a meeting.

Dr. Rodney Johnson, a State Department psychiatrist, visited me twice while I was in the hospital. I thought he was to be my liaison with the State Department. I do not remember what we talked about on his first visit, but on his last visit he hinted that if I could not get to Sri Lanka, my onward assignment, there would be other posts. Bingo. He had nailed my unspoken fear: I would never be able to work again. I would become a burden to my family. I used up that day's allotment of energy insisting that I be allowed to go to Sri Lanka. Weeks later, when I phoned to say I would be leaving the hospital, he explained that I did not have to keep him posted on all my actions. At that point, I realized that he was not a contact person, but someone to consult should I need a psychiatrist. But I had no intention of talking to a psychiatrist within the system. How could I open up to the very person who could pull my medical clearance? I did not want anyone to think that I was not capable of working. Nor did I want to be part of the State Department "corridor gossip." I wanted a normal life.

Certain noises made me jumpy—the backfiring of a car, a firecracker, the dropping of a heavy object. Occasionally I would announce that a bomb had exploded. While in Georgetown Hospital, I informed the nurse on duty that men were firing guns down on the street. I urged her to keep away from the window to avoid being cut by shattering glass. Apparently, it was only the construction workers outside who had dropped some things.

Discharged from the hospital, I rented a house not far from Georgetown Hospital, where I visited daily for several hours of physical therapy. Two nieces, Annie Fitzpatrick and Kathy Dammarell, just out of college, stayed with me that summer. This was a far better alternative to the recommended nursing home. On July 4, 1983, I noted in my journal that I could not sleep that night and walked about thinking someone was outside—or perhaps inside—who wanted to kill me. I felt anxious and had an "inside fear," a deep, new, unnamed fear. I had seen the T.V. program *Cosmos* the previous night. The episode had been on the human brain, which made me ponder the complexity and integration of all things. Knowing that my body had been damaged, I began to speculate that my life might be permanently stunted by the trauma. I was anxious about the brevity of my life and the possibility of my death.

Paradoxically, during this difficult period, my primary emotion was joy. The giddiness and gratitude of being alive filled me. I had seen and heard the pain of others and knew that I was better off than they. I was alive. I had not died. For well over a year, I could not repress my delight.

AID did hold my position for me in Sri Lanka, and I arrived in Colombo in January 1984. When I returned to Washington, D.C., for hand surgery in the summer of 1984, I had irrational fears that someone was going to kill me, and nightmares about being bombed started up. I went to see Margaret Clancy for some tips on how to stop these anxieties. Her advice was to take normal precautions and to talk to my friends, both of which I was doing already. She suggested that I might be having nightmares in the States because I was in a safe place, and felt free to deal with fears which I might suppress in a foreign environment. That seemed reasonable to me. The nightmares stopped.

But disturbing dreams began anew in Sri Lanka, often following violent incidents taking place in that country as its civil war escalated. In May 1984, two American AID contractors working in Jaffna were kidnapped. I did not sleep well until they were released, unharmed, after several days of captivity. A month later, a bomb went off at the Hotel Lanka Oberoi across the street from the Embassy. I was in the Embassy cafeteria eating lunch with a colleague, Eric Lokin. I turned to him and calmly announced that we had just heard a bomb. No one in the cafeteria reacted to my statement. I stayed seated because I did not want to be near the hotel in the case of a second explosion. (In Beirut, a second bomb sometimes would be exploded as people were rescuing the victims of the first blast.) A few minutes later, someone came in and confirmed my suspicion. A couple of days later, our offices were closed so the Marines could do a sweep: the Embassy had received a bomb threat. I began to feel edgy, thinking that the building would be blown up with me in it. I noted in my journal that I wanted to leave Colombo because it was too much like the early days in Beirut. Then the nightmares started. They frequently, but not always, involved bombings. One night I "heard" the loud boom of an explosion which awoke me. I ran to my bedroom window to survey the damage only to realize it was a dream. Since I could understand the relationship between my nightmares and the violence going on in Sri Lanka, I was not particularly concerned.

But when the dreams continued after I was posted in Washington, D.C. in 1986, I was worried enough to visit Dr. Clancy again. I had finally realized that I was not able to will away my fears. The nightmares were always violent and often located in a foreign country. In one I got shot three times on my left side and drove around looking for a hospital, happy to be alive. Another time, my hands were tied behind my back and I was shot in the head by a Philippine death squad. In another, I was back in Beirut in an elevator and one of the two cables snapped. These nightmares became so commonplace that

I could actually tell myself that I was having a "bombing dream" and move on to something else without waking up.

Hypervigilance is not easy to discern once one has lived in Beirut, because lifesaving techniques learned in a war zone are hard to shake, even though they may not be appropriate in another country. When I transferred back to Washington from Sri Lanka, I pulled my desk as far away from the office window as possible as a precaution against flying glass. I figured out the best exits from the State Department. (For a long while, I had to instruct myself to keep walking forward one step at a time, to outfox my apprehension about entering the building.) At home, I ritualistically checked, several times a night, that my doors and windows were locked. I once caused a stir at the local post office when the clerks would not evacuate the building because an unidentified box lay next to the door. I left without buying any stamps.

While at airports, I routinely surveyed people around me to see if they were carrying a bomb. Usually men with briefcases got my most fierce scrutiny. I would stare at the person in front of me, speculating that he or she may be the last person I would ever see. As I became conscious of my exaggerated behavior, I dismissed it as humorous and quirky. Yet when I left AID in 1988, and went to teach in Egypt, whenever possible I avoided walking down the streets where the American Embassy was located. Once I even left the café at the Semiramis Hotel because an elegant American tourist with whom I had struck up a casual conversation had left her purse on her chair next to mine when she went to select a pastry. She seemed to be taking too long at the dessert buffet and I began fantasizing that she had planted a bomb in her purse.

While I was teaching at a Coptic Catholic seminary in Alexandria, Egypt, in 1988, a small, chemical factory next door blew up, causing a fire. At 2:15 a.m., I awoke to shouts of *"Allah Akbar"*[31] and saw sheets of flames though the glass section of my bedroom door. My first thought as I leapt from my bed was, "How did they know I was here?" Believing we had been bombed, I prepared to jump out my window to escape the fire and the expected second blast. Concrete, not grass, covered the ground below my third floor window. On second thought, I opened my bedroom door to exit to the back garden for safety.

Struggling to put the bombing episode behind me as if it were a burnt pot roast, an unappetizing reality not to be dwelt upon, I resolved that it would not dominate my life. Had anyone told me that I was in denial, I would have laughed. I consciously did everything I could to deal with the trauma of the bombing in a productive fashion.

Not being able to mourn the deaths of my colleagues and my absolute lack of interest in the driver who detonated the bomb were early clues that something was amiss, but I did not consider them avoidance symptoms. I understood from the start that the nightmares, interrupted sleeping patterns, and inside fears were related to Beirut, and yet I chastised myself for not being able to "get over them and get on with life," as though the explosion was a nettlesome gnat.

Upon reflection, I now see that some of my thoughts and behavior were forms of denial. I believed that I should not talk "too much" about the bombing for fear of making the story trivial chit-chat. At times I felt that I was describing a third person, not myself. For a long while I was convinced that only my fellow-survivor Bob Pearson could understand the experience. Prior to his death in 1991, Bob and I often discussed Beirut and the impact that the bombing had had on our lives. His death was a great loss to me.

Not writing about my experience may have been another form of denial. Marsha Darling, a history professor at Georgetown University, suggested that writing this thesis would be part of the healing process for me. She was right. The Air Force doctor who examined me in the plane en route to Wiesbaden was the first to suggest that I write up my experience. Nine years later, in 1992, I started. Then, for no conscious reason, I stopped. This thesis has given me an incentive to continue that process.

The explosion has made a difference in my life, and yet my life has not altered dramatically. Thinking in superlatives, my strongest conscious emotional response to Beirut was—and is—joy. The bombing gave me an appreciation of life for which I am grateful. While the high of being alive lasted for only a year, I am still conscious of being alive and being able to walk, conditions I took for granted prior to 1983. For several years, I was preoccupied with the notion that my life had been spared for one specific purpose. The burden of playing Dick Tracy to discover my "task" weighed me down until I saw the folly of my thinking. A near-death experience does not superimpose special responsibilities, but rather gives a heightened appreciation of life. My perception of life, its brevity and purpose, still gives me pause. I still believe we humans are to live our lives as fully as possible while being of service to others, and I still fear death.

While in the hospital, my deepest frustration was rooted in being physically helpless and totally dependent on others. My greatest motive for regaining health was the desire to be able to work again. My most secret fear was that I would never be "normal" again.

After I had returned to Washington, a friend mentioned that I might have post- traumatic stress disorder. I dismissed his comment because I *knew* that PTSD was what soldiers went through, not civilians. PTSD was serious. All that I had to contend with was a memory of a bombing.

I kept a journal while living overseas. For this paper, I reviewed my journals dating from 1983 through 1987 to determine if any of my comments indicated symptoms of post- traumatic stress disorder. They did. By cross-referencing the symptoms of post-traumatic stress disorder with the notes in my journals, I concluded that there was a match. Until writing this paper, I had not understood that I had experienced post-traumatic stress disorder. I found it comforting to have a model to hang my symptoms on. I liked knowing that my responses were similar to those of other victims of trauma.

I would have benefited from talking in specific terms about the predictable response to trauma in the early stages of recovery. Such information would have lessened my apprehension about not being normal. I felt that information was being withheld from me when I tried to get a this-is-what-is-going-to-happen outline from the psychiatrists. I had the impression that they thought I would copycat the symptoms. I just wanted to be prepared.

It would have been useful to have trusted the system enough to have felt free to consult with the State Department Medical Center, assuming they had staff trained in dealing with post-traumatic stress disorder. The Foreign Service is different from other types of work. Talking with people who serve overseas does make a difference, since we all have had similar experiences and share a common language. I would have benefited had I been contacted by State Medical after I had recuperated and been told about the aftermath reactions to terrorist attacks. They would have had to contact me, since I was too ignorant and scared to contact them.

Postscript: After writing this section of the thesis, I met with Dr. Clancy to ask her what her diagnosis of me had been in 1988. She laughed when I said I had met with her once before leaving for Sri Lanka. I had visited fifteen times. I nodded when she said she had diagnosed me as having post-traumatic stress disorder.

Chapter 4

FOREIGN SERVICE OFFICERS' RECOLLECTIONS

A   INTERVIEWS WITH FSOs

In addition to the military, forty-four Foreign Service Officers survived the bombing. Fourteen FSOs were interviewed for this study. I met individually with the eight who lived in the Washington, D.C., area and telephoned the remaining six. The interviews ranged from one to three hours. Of the fourteen, five were men and nine were women. Eight were retired and six were still in the Foreign Service.

Nine had worked for the State Department, four for the Agency for International Development, and one for the United States Information Service at the time of the explosion. Their length of service ranged from two to thirty-two years. For all but three, Beirut had been either the first or second posting in the Middle East. Although none immediately left Beirut because of the bombing, three said that they would not be willing to return. (One left the Foreign Service because of the U.S. policy in the Middle East.) Most had accepted the assignment because the State Department or a previous supervisor personally asked them to go. Three actively sought the assignment to get out of their previous postings. Two volunteered because they had friends in Lebanon.

Eight were injured. One broke her toe jumping from the Embassy. Seven got cut by flying glass during the explosion. Some required stitches. None was hospitalized.

I conducted the telephone interviews first. The interviews by phone differed somewhat from those conducted face-to-face. The phone sessions tended to be briefer and explanations of the long-term impact of the incident less philosophical. These differences could be a reflection of my "newness" in conducting the interviews or the lack of personal contact. The only other significant difference was that all with whom I met personally felt that the State Department gave them sufficient support following the bombing. Three of the six with whom I spoke by phone felt that they did not receive sufficient support.

Foreign Service Officers' Immediate Reaction to Bombing

Virtually all who were alive in 1963 can recall where they were when they learned of President Kennedy's assassination. In similar fashion, all in this sample knew the details of where they were when dynamite blasted away the Embassy in 1983.

Several feared a follow-up explosion. As anyone living in Lebanon at that time knew, a second bomb designed to detonate about fifteen minutes after the first often killed many targeted victims along with rescue workers. "Everybody get down, there could be a second one," were the first words that Ryan Crocker remembered saying. Barbara Gregory thought that she was back in Cambodia: "I was on my hands and knees trying to get under the equipment because I thought...we're going to be hit again with a rocket." Tish Butler felt a need to escape because she thought the gas tanks stored in the building would explode.

Sudden and unexpected, the loud blast jolted everyone even though not everyone heard the explosion. "It just happened. You didn't know if it was an earthquake or a bomb from the sky. It was just so fast and unexpected," said Dorothy Pech. Yet Ambassador Robert Dillon and Christine Crocker did not hear a sound. Crocker only felt the heat of hot wind sliding across the back of her head, which had been forced down against her desk. As the brick wall blew out very slowly and collapsed across him, Dillon thought, "My God, those so-and-so's almost got me that time."

The lack of a staircase or front wall and piles of rubble made exiting difficult. Few understood the extent of the damage until they tried to make their way out. Most remained calm, a reaction which facilitated getting the wounded out.

As Ryan Crocker recounted,

> I was, and all those aro5und me were, extremely calm, including those injured. Time seemed to move in very, very slow motion. A very methodical process of looking after the injured and moving people out got underway...The enormity of what had happened was

clear because that [Post One[32]] was like walking into hell. It was pitch black. The face of the building had collapsed in on the lobby and fires were burning inside. It was very clear that no one in that area could possibly have survived.

Gregory recalled,

It was so eerie. It really was. No noise. No nothing. I would come down a few steps and stop and listen. I thought everybody was dead but me. I had forgotten about seeing all my friends running out and thought, "I'm the only one alive." But anyway, it was really traumatic. I went into this shock type thing and I just sort of stayed that way.

Faith Lee claimed that, "It was like we were all zombies."

Several commented on seeing friends and colleagues who were hurt, and assisting them to escape. Butler talked of seeing Mary Lee McIntyre, wife of the AID Deputy Director, whose face had been cut by flying glass. "Blood was pooled up in her eyes and streaming down her white, white face." Gregory noted that Mary Apovian "had been scalped and the blood was so thick that you could hardly see the tip of her nose." To get out of the Embassy compound,

Dick Gannon said, he and

one of the military men bent the gate and grillwork back as far as we could so that people could crawl out over and climb down the wall at the back of the Chancery into a dirt field. I helped a number of people who had lined up to come out of the Embassy.

Dazed at the time, Beth Samuel stated that "to this day I don't remember Dennis Foster, but he says that he helped lift me over the fence to the ambulance. I guess I was just totally in shock because even now I don't remember it."

Rikkie Smith reflected the thinking of others as she described instructing herself: "I became very clearheaded and thought, I must be helpful. I must not panic. I must not act scared. I must not throw up."

Diane Dillard consciously deferred thinking about the loss of life of colleagues and friends. "When I went around to the front of the building for the first time, I could see a great hunk of my section was gone. Two-thirds of my office was gone. I thought, well, I'll have to think about that later."

Many were concerned about notifying family members in the States. "The main thing was to get to my apartment to call my family to tell them I was o.k.," Lee said. A friend of Samuel's, "Annalisa Meyer, bless her, called my mother. She saved my parents a tremendous amount of trauma by telling them before they saw it on T.V. My husband was driving to work and heard it on the radio." Kurt Shafer "went back to the apartment and called my parents. They were watching it all on T.V. and quite obviously relieved to hear that I was fine."

Dave Mandel could not contact his children immediately:

> One way or another most of them found out about it through the news. All they heard was that the Embassy was blown up. They had to wait several hours before they found out whether we were safe or not. It was very hard on them, particularly our younger son, who at the time was twelve or thirteen.

Most spoke of putting all of their energy into work. As Samuel explained, the Deputy Chief of Mission "Bob Pugh had a meeting at 8:30 the next morning, and it never occurred to anyone not to go. I don't think it occurred to anybody not to get up and go to work. You felt better being there." As Ambassador Dillon recalled, "You're so busy doing what you're doing that you don't have time to reflect on the horror. I think that's what happened to all of us." Ryan Crocker agreed. "Various chemical reactions tended to keep us calm, carrying us straight through, dovetailing with exhaustion. We went several nights without sleep, supervising the search and recovery of bodies." Sleep became a luxury for some. When John Reid told Dillard that he had only got five hours of sleep, she thought, "[F]ive hours sleep, how wonderful!...I was exhausted...I did not really recover from the whole experience of Beirut while I was there."

Mandel said that AID was functioning "and back in business after a couple of days. I was just really busy with that. You don't stop and think about things. You just keep going."

Lee told of returning to

> her office to make sure I got all of my classified [material] out. But the building wasn't really good for a whole lot of walking and carrying things up and down, but I was responsible. I was responsible for all the classified materials. I was very conscientious about my job....

Gregory also returned to the Embassy:

> I had to go back in three days later and that distressed me something terribly [sic]. I had to lead the Marines and our people in. They were going up to get the equipment out and they didn't know how to get up there. There was nobody to show them, so I had to go back into the Embassy and climb up to the sixth floor. I could feel the floors shaking. I was very, very nervous about it when I was up there.

While a few specifically wanted to be alone, others were afraid to be. Smith wanted to stay home the next day "to think about the bombing. I wanted to relive things to see what I could remember, because you do block out a lot of things immediately." Dillard "needed to be alone to try to come to grips with things." However, Christine Crocker remembered "being absolutely terrified to be home by myself. It took me the longest time to get over. I don't think it left me for a long time, even when we were back in the States." Pech said that for "the first time I could not be alone." She stayed with the Pughs for several days.

A few FSOs mentioned having nightmares. Smith claimed to be:

> a nightmare person...I have such dreams that I wonder where they are coming from...but I don't relive the bombing anymore. I've gotten that out of my mind somehow. I thought I would be reliving it for a year, but I wasn't. I would say in four to six months it was gone. Almost the memory of it was gone.

One night Gannon found himself "startled awake and pushing the blankets off...I felt I was buried under something." He attributes that to having spent one week digging through rubble and lifting up slabs of concrete in search of victims.

One of the roughest tasks was to identify the bodies sent to the morgue at the American University Hospital (AUH). Dillard spent a lot of time at the morgue and "must have sent my nose on vacation" because she wasn't bothered by the smell until months later, when she returned to talk to one of the workers at the morgue. She then wondered how she had managed that first week following the bombing.

> Butler spent between three and five minutes in the morgue. That was the worst part of the whole event for me. It seared images of bodies and body parts on my consciousness, which stuck with me for a while...For a couple of months I saw these images...and would have to forcefully, willfully put them out of my mind.

Although most spoke of working hard and in harmony with others, a few references were made to being irritable because of the strain of the bombing. Learning that a meeting had been called, and that she had not been one of the first informed, Dorothy Pascoe said that "I really lit into Pugh when I found that out. I really let him have it both barrels when I got to his place. Here I am the Ambassador's secretary and nobody was calling me. I was really ticked off."

Christine Crocker recalled a party weeks later where tempers flared late in the evening:

> People did feel a little bit more tense about their lives... No one talked about the bombing until late in the evening when they had too much to drink...People got angry with each other for a while. It blew up. They never said anything specific. I think it was a reaction. People, mostly the Marines, were just angry.

Most found comfort in talking to colleagues. Pech noted that she "talked more. Talking helps. Talk with colleagues, people who can understand. It's no good with others." When Dillard went to England as part of her R&R, one of the British employees who had lived in London during World War II sat her down and asked to be told all about Beirut. Dillard said, "It was wonderful talking with someone who knew about death and dying...It would have been nice to talk with someone in the Department, but I didn't know anyone. No one sought me out."

Gregory claimed that:

> It has never, never left me...It's embedded in my brain and I don't usually talk about it. Of course, I don't talk about it to people in Florida. People in Florida don't understand our lifestyle. They really don't. I've told some of them. Once in a while we get into it. It's usually when another Foreign Service person comes that I talk to them. If they haven't been overseas and lived our life, they don't understand it.

Samuel said,

> the only thing that I feel a little bit guilty about is that I didn't have any desire to be home or to talk to my family or to talk to my husband. I felt that these [colleagues] were the people I wanted to be with right now. They [the psychiatrists] told me that was very normal.

Dillon stressed the importance of spouses sharing danger. It was important personally that Sue and I have shared a lot of the danger in Lebanon. It made it far easier for me to adjust after that [Beirut] than after some experiences during the Korean war, which I didn't share with anybody. I always had the feeling my family never understood.

Butler agreed that her experience would have been very different had she not been posted with her husband. "Malcolm was very [supportive]. I don't remember whether he asked a lot of questions or whether he just was there to listen when I needed help, but he was my sounding board."

A few mentioned being asked about Beirut at social gatherings. Smith said that, "A lot of people talked to you just sort of out of the blue. You were a celebrity for a while." Mandel mentioned the "cocktail talk," stressing that he doesn't "really talk about it much."

Butler noted that

> it was an almost inexpressible experience. What I ran into was a lot of people asking questions to which there could either be a ten-word answer or a two-hour answer. Most of the time I gave a ten-word answer. I

felt like it required too much to go into to really convey the real feelings and the real experience.

Most mentioned the first time they cried. Each person had a different time frame. For Christine Crocker, it was the early hours of the day after the bombing. "They were still getting people out and we were there all night. Then the Marines raised the flag. Probably that was when I first cried." For Dillon, it was about a week or ten days later in the American University of Beirut (AUB) chapel as he addressed the Lebanese families of those who had died. "I was down to about the last sentence or two and I just couldn't go on...I just stopped. That was the first time I really felt emotionally overwhelmed by the bombing."

For Pech,

> [i]t wasn't until six weeks later when I was home. I went down to Texas where my son was graduating from college...I started to tell him about something. I barely could talk and I felt so stupid, but the tears started coming.

For Samuel

> when the five-year mark came...[a friend] said something about what happened five years ago...I started crying and I cried and I cried and I cried and I cried. Even now when I talk to people I feel tears, whereas I didn't the first couple of years after it happened. I guess I was just in denial or blocking it out.

Several believed living through the experience made them stronger. Butler remembered "feeling very shaken but very strong at the same time. I remember feeling that I had to hold it together, that I could because I was o.k." Christine Crocker felt "pretty good" about herself because she did not fall to pieces which was "reassuring...It is funny because I would think, how could I have known that if I hadn't been there."

Samuel said,

> I did find that I was much stronger than I ever would have thought. Going to work the next morning, pitching in, helping set up offices and going to see the families of the people who died—I just automatically

did these things, because I knew they had to be done. I never would have thought that I would be strong enough to do that.

Two had a strong desire to return to Lebanon as a way of resolving their emotional reactions to the bombing. Lee asserted that while in Japan, her assignment after Lebanon, ...

> every time I talked about the bombing and the people I had seen hurt, I would start crying, and even talking to her [the psychiatrist] I would start crying. The one thing I felt within me was to get back to Beirut. I had to get back to see it for myself and see some of the people. She didn't advise it. About three months later, I requested to volunteer to go to Beirut. I went back in May or April of 1984 for TDY. I saw some of the people. I had lunch with Mary Apovian. I met and talked to some of the other people. I was there a month. Now I feel better. This healed me. When I went back to Tokyo, I could talk about the bombing. Now I can talk about it. I don't cry. This was my way of knowing I could be healed.

Pech also felt that returning to Beirut after her home leave was "absolutely the best psychological therapy."

Impact of Bombing on Foreign Service Officers

Many placed the bombing of the Embassy within the context of war. Although devastating for some, it was not the only, or even the worst, experience in Beirut. The horror of the massacre of hundreds of Palestinian civilians in Sabra-Shatila[33] in the fall of 1982 was most frequently cited. For Christine Crocker, "Sabra-Shatila was almost worse [than the bombing]." Kurt Shafer cautioned: "One must remember that there were a series of things in Beirut, and really and truly the shelling sometimes was a lot more frightening than the actual incident at the Embassy was."

For Butler,

> April 18, 1983, was less traumatic for me than the shelling of West Beirut in late August, early September [of that year]. I had much more sustained susceptibility

> to death. Shells were landing around us for thirty-six hours, and also I was feeling more mortal because of what we had gone through three months before…

Dillard remarked that "[t]he bombing was the worst thing that happened to the Embassy family, but it wasn't the end of crisis. Everyday was kind of a crisis. We were shelled a lot. <u>The</u> bombing was like the beginning." Dillon noted that "[t]he bombing was a very dramatic incident, and on one level I'm still angry. But, I can't say that I was emotionally any more bothered by that than I was over Sabra-Shatila."

Pascoe

> was more frightened when we were evacuated at the Ambassador's residence. Because those RPGs were coming around the Ambassador's so much. We used to go outside and stand on the patio and watch everything that was going on. It was horrible. Well, the residence did get hit in a couple of places, but not badly. I really was a little more frightened then, than after the bombing of the Embassy.

Ryan Crocker

> put the bombing in the larger frame of events in Lebanon…as bad as it was, it wasn't the only event: the Israeli invasion itself, the Sabra-Shatila massacres, the attempted takeover of West Beirut by the militia in 1983…The bombing became a part of rather a long three-year time of trial.

Butler wrestled with

> a little bit of survivor's guilt…I was absolutely consumed with trying to figure out, which of course was impossible, why I left the cafeteria early that day, why I was healthy and others were dead…It seemed to me that there should have been more beneficial knowledge coming out of that experience than came.

Butler also talked about being "intent on being all right afterwards…at that time it was important for me to feel that I was o.k. So I didn't dwell on it and didn't want to dwell on it." Dillon mentioned that he felt normal and asked the psychiatrist if something were wrong with him. "The guy told me these were normal reactions because psychologically we put up defenses or we couldn't live through these things. They would destroy us."

Although several said that the bombing did not change their lives, others mentioned that it gave them a heightened appreciation of life. Smith felt the "next day everything seemed so precious, every little thing was so particularly special that you notice it. You don't take anything for granted for a long time, and then you start flipping back into your old ways."

Butler said,

> For most of my life, I have tried to figure out what I believe about God and why we're here. I sort of honed my interest in figuring it out and also just absolutely reveled in being here. For the next six or seven years, I chose to live my life trying to make the most of it.

According to Ryan Crocker, people cannot "live through something like the bombing without having it affect them. It certainly made me very glad to be alive."

Both Dillon and Ryan Crocker use the bombing as a measuring rod. As expressed by Dillon, "Occasionally, when Sue and I are discouraged about something, we look at each other and say, 'Well, what the hell, we're alive.'"

> Several talked of becoming aware of their own mortality. Gannon believes that … it certainly has made me more aware of my own vulnerability in terms of emotional vulnerability…This particular event in my life really showed me that you're not quite as tough as you might have envisioned that you were. A lot of wonderful, productive people died that afternoon… When someone goes through something as traumatic as that, you tend to reflect back and ask many questions which have possibly no answers, or at least the answers are not available to us. But, it does have an effect in terms of seeing your own mortality. You see your own vulnerability.

Several maintained that they overreacted to subsequent noise or news about Lebanon. Some still do. Lee said, "The bombing made me more alert. When I first came home, I would hear a car backfire, I was like jumping, but I got over that." Gregory was in the lobby of a hotel in Spain when she learned about the Marine barracks being hit.

> ...I went totally hysterical and I embarrassed myself to the point where I went upstairs and didn't go back out...It's just I hated the violence and how it affects me. I was never afraid of thunderstorms or lightning. Now I can't take any loud noises anymore. Thunder makes me so very nervous. Thunderstorms, that's where I notice it the most, because I used to love them....But Beirut changed everything. My sister on our trip to Spain that fall [1983] dropped a window in one of our rooms, and I came tearing out of the bed and my heart was going five million miles an hour. It was just terrible, terrible. It affects everybody. I don't know how anyone could go through something like that and not be affected.

Shafer declared that,

> Loud noises in Beirut sort of bothered one, but it was more from the bombing all of the time rather than from that one incident. If there were a loud explosion or loud bang, a firecracker, a car backfiring, it seemed like I jumped a little higher than usual. That lasted a few years, but I haven't jumped in a few years. Loud noises really did use to scare the daylights out of me.

Many talked about an increased awareness of security issues and how the nature of the Foreign Service has changed as a result of the escalation of terrorism. Lee said that the bombing "...made me more suspicious...it just made me know that you cannot trust, you cannot let your guard down, especially if you're in a post overseas." Ryan Crocker noted that,

> Going back to Beirut as Ambassador, one rather obvious goal I set for myself was that we would not be the object of a car bomb or any other major attack. We

would have every means whatsoever of preventing it and be extremely methodical in going over our security.

When Crocker briefs new Foreign Service Officers, he tells them that

> ... virtually every single officer in the room, if she or he pursues a fifteen-or twenty-year stint in the State Department (assuming that they don't spend it all in Western Europe), would see, almost without doubt, shots fired in anger, witness an evacuation in some form or other—dependents or personnel—and would be in a crisis of some magnitude. That is simply the way of the world.

Dillard declared that,

> When I went to Florence in the fall of 1985, I was very concerned about the building, because our building in Beirut had been so vulnerable. In Italy, we were right on the street. I finally got the Embassy in Rome and the City Government to let us put up a barrier. Once that happened, then I forgot about it. I had done all I could do to protect the building and employees. But until then, I was always sure I was going to come around the corner and see it blow up.

Mandel said that:

> Since I've been in Beirut, I find that most missions overseas base their briefing of new people on the current level of threats. Everybody's perception is that the post is real safe. They don't really worry about emergency evacuation plans or whatever. I think that's a mistake because things can change pretty quickly and if people aren't prepared before, then you run into problems. I think there needs to be a greater emphasis in overseas missions. In Washington, they have this course [Security Overseas Seminar] and they think it is fine. When you get to post, emergency evacuation plans, bomb preparedness plans, who's responsible for what, that sort of stuff, should be run through with people.

> But it isn't done. They are supposed to be briefing the newcomers but it doesn't take place. People tend to avoid [it]. It's a real problem. They say, it can't happen here. It's very safe. A safe post tends to get a little sloppy and it's hard to get people to keep their guards up. I tend to say, the people who have experienced the full consequences of not keeping their guard up are more inclined to take precautions.

Dillon is

> troubled, indeed saddened, by the defenses behind which our people live. Embassies look like giant prisons. They're big fortresses. Isolated. And yet I remind myself that if we had had something like that in Lebanon, we would have been secure. Secure and they could not have blown up the Embassy. If anyone wants to pursue a Foreign Service life, this is part of it. It's like being in the Army. There isn't any safe way to do it.

Gannon believes that a serious issue which

> people who have joined the Foreign Service must accept [is]...that they may be putting themselves, possibly their families, at increased risk, simply because they are representing the United States Government abroad. Are they willing to accept that? I think each individual needs to weigh that very carefully, because you do not have the guarantees abroad—even if you are carrying that diplomatic passport—that we basically have here in the States.

A few spoke of the lasting effect of the bombing, while others asserted that they were not frightened by the bombing and that it had little impact on their lives. Gregory described her feelings: "All I did was feel this horrible, horrible sorrow that somebody could do this to innocent people and their own people. You never get over something like that. It's something I've never gotten over." Yet Pascoe mentioned that:

> I don't think I was frightened at all. I really, honestly, to this day, I don't think I was ever frightened. I think

I was more excited, the old adrenaline starts pumping away. I know it was horrible, but I certainly wasn't scared. I was really more excited about "My God, what's going to happen next?" The bombing didn't make any difference in my life. I look back, of course. Many people ask, "Oh, you were in Beirut, were you there during the bombing?" I have to go through this whole thing with them, where I was, how I felt, and the whole thing. It's about the only time I really think about it. I mean, I remember that I was there and what happened. Sure, I think about it. Not in a bad way, because I tell everybody that I really enjoyed my tour while I was over there, and I did! I really did enjoy my tour with everything that was going on. When you go into the Foreign Service, as far as I'm concerned, you've got to expect something like this. Particularly in these volatile type countries.

Shafer stated that, "I reckon it's the single most trying experience I've had, but it was not all that traumatic, all that life-threatening. More in the mind. A natural threat of damage to the person."

Christine Crocker caught the sentiment of more than one interviewee when she mused that the bombing of the Embassy is

one of those events that you think about on a fairly regular basis and for an unknown reason, I don't know why. It's something I think about a lot. I don't know how to change that. Deep down change that. I can't tell you exactly why. I don't think it's made me a better person. I know that if it ever happened to me [again], I could still carry on.

Views on Why the Embassy was Bombed

When asked for an opinion as to why the Embassy was bombed, most cited a combination of U.S. policy in the Middle East and inadequate security procedures, while others only cited one of the two reasons. Some had held the belief that as Americans they would be invulnerable. Lee explained why she felt invulnerable.

> I didn't think that anybody was going to hurt me. I wasn't an enemy, so I felt free walking the streets. I never felt threatened. I never felt that they were going to pick me out of a crowd and get me...We got too carefree. That's what it was, and we let our guard down.

Others believed differently. Dillard stated simply "...they were trying to kill the Ambassador, because he was the symbol of America." Dillon outlined his views in greater detail.

> We were targeted by the Shiite group, Hizballah. It was the Musawi family over in the Bekaa that apparently did it. The Shiites were outraged by the Israeli invasion of Lebanon. They were outraged that they were in the hands of the Israelis. They saw us as the pillar of support, going along with all of these people. They believed that perhaps we had put the Israelis up to the invasion, which, of course, we didn't. On the other hand, we did foolish things. After the invasion, Congress voted to increase military aid to the Israelis. They [Hizballah] decided that we were their enemies. The idea of a blow against the greatest nation in the world was something that appealed to them very strongly and something that people were willing to give their lives for, and they did. The idea that the downtrodden could inflict major injury on the greatest power on earth was very important.

The other thing that had happened on the ground was that physically we had lost our defenses. The PLO and the Druze militia protected us, not for humanitarian reasons, but for political reasons. They had a stake in our presence. I think we were slow to understand the consequences of having been shorn of all that protection and that we were on our own resources. We were very vulnerable. We understood that. There had been car bombs all over the place. We reacted to that. We had cleared out the area around the Embassy. A car couldn't stop, for instance, and an abandoned car was destroyed. The possibility of a suicide attack was understood and we had ordered some barriers to be put up. Some ram-proof barriers had just arrived but weren't up.

There is another level—it makes you sound like a boob—but there is another level at which you don't realize how vulnerable you really are. Americans can and do engage in suicidal attacks [in terms of disregarding danger]. This is part of our culture. You realize that your chances of being killed are very high on a suicidal attack. We don't engage in suicide attacks [i.e., t]he kamikaze idea is just so foreign to our culture that we talk about it in the abstract. It's no longer abstract, but in 1983 a suicide attack was a very abstract idea still. We had one example, and we weren't even sure of that. The Iraqi Embassy was destroyed.

Nobody knew what had happened, but we speculated that it had been a suicide attack. The first time we really knew that these people, in fact, would engage in suicide attacks was when our Embassy was destroyed.

I understand that the Musawi backed by the Iranians were involved. I don't know that anybody had any information to directly implicate the Syrians; on the other hand, neither the Musawis nor the Iranians could have operated without at least Syrian acquiescence, because both operated right out of Syrian-controlled Bekaa.

Ryan Crocker gave a similar explanation for why the Embassy was taken by surprise:

> It hadn't happened before. It is very difficult to understand what may happen to you if you don't have some kind of experiential base to deal with, and massive suicide bomb attacks on American embassies just simply were not part of the inventory.

Gannon discussed the security issue specifically:

> I don't feel that anyone foresaw the situation being as dangerous as it was...I knew that security at the site and in the building were probably not what you might have had at other embassies. There were reasons for that, and certainly the administrative officer and I had discussed that. His views were, we don't want to sink a lot of money into this building because we might not [continue to] be here. We've had to leave it once or twice, and so we're really trying to be reasonable about

this. That was his perspective. But looking back, should we have had a perimeter fence around us? Sure, we certainly should have. I recall someone before the blast coming out from Washington and was there specifically to review the security in place. He said, "This is well below any sort of standard that we would have for any U.S. government facility overseas." That was his viewpoint. My view was, give me some money and we'll do whatever we can do with the money we have. At that time, there was no security budget as such. The money wasn't allocated that way. It was regional bureau money or post money that security improvements were made from, and the post understandably did not want to expend a lot of money if it was going to be wasted. [In a March 16 follow-up call, Gannon clarified that provisions for a fence were made a month before the bombing. His disappointment was "that it was not in October when we settled back in West Beirut, rather than in February or March 1983."]

Preparation for Danger Posts

For most, the only preparation for a danger post was a one-day course, "Coping with Violence Abroad," offered to all FSOs going overseas. Only three of the Foreign Service Officers interviewed had been in the military. It can be assumed that their experience better prepared them for the bombing than those without military service. Several mentioned experiences in other hardship posts. A few Foreign Service Officers felt that they were not adequately prepared for facing a terrorist attack and that no amount of training could have prepared them. A few mentioned how much more helpful the newer "Security Overseas Seminar" was than the previous "Coping with Violence Abroad" course, which did not directly deal with bombings or the effects of terrorist activities. Smith recalled that, "Years before, I had something called 'evasive' training. It was like counter-terrorism training. They taught us how to evade if someone was trying to push us off the road." Samuel thought that

> none of us had had any preparation for something like that [the bombing]. I know I had not. The only thing

> that USIS tried to get you to do was to take defensive driving, which was ridiculous. First of all, you couldn't have a car in Beirut. It would have been ridiculous anyway, because all they had to do was shoot you. I don't think that there was any preparation for the psychological effect of being without your spouse or living for months on end in a hotel.

Butler remembered that

> when I did attend, ["Coping with Violence Abroad"] was all focused on kidnapping and hostage situations and nothing particularly relevant to that bombing experience. As a matter of fact, I think the bombing experience turned around and formed the rethinking of that course a little bit. I don't feel that I had any formal preparation for [the bombing].

Butler also believed that "people [should] know in advance some basics about what they should expect in terms of their own personal reactions, their own human reactions to trauma."

Mandel said that the Security Overseas Seminar has been improving over the years. "I took it six or seven years ago, and I think they do a pretty good job of briefing people." Christine Crocker agreed. "I think the two-day briefing is a good course, and I really do think that people in this day have to keep aware."

At the request of the overseas missions, the Department of State made several videos dealing with traumatic aspects of living overseas as Foreign Service Officers. Because of her experience as Chief of the Consular Section at the time of the bombing, Dillard was interviewed for the video "Crisis Work, Crisis Worker." She felt that making the training video was very good for her.

> Before I went to Florence [for my next assignment], I talked to Sheila Platt.[34] When I came back for the filming, I also spent a lot of time with Marilyn Holmes,[35] hours discussing things. I was a little worried about it before I started the filming. I hadn't really talked about those things with anybody. In the filming, Sheila would bring up things that I had said to her the

summer before and that I had forgotten. I realized that actually I was getting over it and putting it behind me. It was very positive for me to get to do that. I shared my feelings, because I thought that would be helpful to other people. It wasn't until I saw the tape in the fall of 1985 that I understood what I had experienced was a type of shock. They called it denial, a stress reaction. Denial is an all right kind of stress reaction to have. I was glad to know that was not unique to me.

Ryan Crocker has concluded that there are two things needed to prepare Foreign Service Officers for life overseas:

> First is, make people aware of the fact that new world order is very much new world disorder in terms of threat, and that they have to think about it and take responsibility for thinking about it. They can't simply look to other forces or elements to protect them from danger. But the second thing is, to mitigate that by making it simply part of our life, not to scare people with it, but to go over it so often that it becomes normal, so that people are not frightened by the idea of thinking about risk and threat and danger. Part of our overseas role should be to de-mystify danger...

Gannon stressed the need for personal anticipatory reflection and informed decision making. He believed that the

> Department prepares the Foreign Service personnel as well as they can be prepared for the great unknown... You don't have the protection. I think the Department has gone a long way in terms of briefing programs, addressing these types of issues, and certainly the Department and Congress have gone a long way in trying to put security resources in the right locales. But then again terrorism is not something that is easily contained. We no sooner build a secure facility in one country, and we have an incident pop up in another country. The Department has sponsored, with a great deal of effort and money, crisis management exercises

for Washington and at high-threat posts. It certainly is something that we did not have in Beirut. It's probably a credit to the leadership in Beirut. People really did a magnificent job, I think, given the circumstances and given the fact that they never had any rehearsal. Today, many posts have had the opportunity to have a rehearsal and they should be that much better equipped to address these types of tragedies.

Follow-up Support After the Bombing

The State Department provided support to the FSOs in Beirut at the time of the bombing. The regional medical doctor posted in Cairo flew directly to Beirut, and two psychiatrists were sent to talk to the staff. Some FSOs found the visits useful. Others did not. Some did not talk with the doctors, because they felt no need to do so, while others did not meet with the medical personnel because they did not respect the field of psychiatry or psychiatrists from the State Department. In addition, a special Rest and Recuperation (R&R) trip to Washington was authorized for those permanently assigned to Lebanon.

Dillard reported that,

> A psychiatrist came on the plane from Washington. I assume he talked to everybody. He talked to me. I know that he talked to some others. I enjoyed talking to him. It was helpful to me. He had a very commonsense approach. A couple of weeks after that, they sent another psychiatrist in to talk to groups and individuals.

Smith talked to a psychiatrist who "was terrific. She made us all talk about our feelings and fears and our wants and our needs. The psychiatrist wanted us to talk a lot about the bombing, in case we still had something we were blocking up inside."

Ryan Crocker noted that

> [w]e were all encouraged, indeed directed, to see her. She was very pleasant, very level-headed. She was good in the sense that she was not demanding that you unveil a crisis to her. If you were feeling o.k., it was

fine with her. I had a very brief conversation with her. Generally speaking, I thought it was nice that they sent in a psychiatrist. I didn't really feel the need then or afterwards to talk to one.

Butler mentioned that they

> tried to schedule everybody for half an hour interviews. I certainly don't remember it being a lifesaving experience. I think they needed to do that, and maybe some people benefitted more. I think there could have been a little more done. There could have been more gathering together as a family, letting feelings out as a family and as a group. In the Philippines they actually brought in In-Touch Foundation, a local organization, private volunteer organization staffed with psychiatrists and clinical social workers. They actually brought them in to deal with the post-traumatic feelings. That was more effective than a visit from one regional psychiatrist.

Samuel felt that the psychiatric support was

> just a big farce and we kind of hooted about it later. Somebody said, "I think they learned a lot talking to us." By the time they brought them in, it was too late. We had all done our crying. We had had each other as therapy. That's what everyone talked about for days and days.

Gannon recalled that

> [e]veryone had an appointed time to go see the doctor and just sort of talk through how they were doing. At the appointed time, I showed up, knocked on the door, and the doctor was still dealing with the person ahead of me and asked if we could reschedule. I said, "Certainly." I had things to do anyway, and to be quite honest with you, I never really got back. The Department did the correct thing. I think having somebody with professional qualifications come on the scene like that is very helpful. It gives people someone to go to, to cope with that type of trauma.

Christine Crocker had intended "to talk to the psychiatrist, but it was just one of those things. I just ended up not having time. People got their lives back to normal as quickly as they could and did what they could..."

Pech "chose not to talk to them. I suppose they must have thought, 'Oh! she's one of those.' I was handling this myself. I didn't have anything to say. I had to work through it. I was fine. It worked out. I worked through by working and talking to friends". Pech added "What is a psychiatrist? I don't care if he has twenty degrees, you feel sort of silly...like what does he understand; it's got to be your colleagues. I don't like to talk to them [Foreign Service psychiatrists] too much."

Pascoe felt that the bombing

> didn't really affect me all that much. I don't know if I'm a strong personality, or what. I was crushed that so many people and friends were killed, but personally it didn't bother me. It really didn't. We had the psychiatrist there and I didn't need to talk to her because I didn't need to.

Mandel thought that a lot of people did not go to see the psychiatrists.

> This was ten years ago and we were learning a lot of things at that time. I don't think that the people in the business really understood all of the ramifications. I don't think the State Department at that stage was all that sensitive and concerned. I mean they were: "Just get on with the business, and if you need help, it's there." It's not like now: when you get some sort of really traumatic experience, they send in whole teams. They have organized activities and they say, "Everybody will come and we'll talk." It's much more aggressive, because people like me are very introspective. My tendency is to withdraw into myself. Far as I know I did fine. I didn't have any real problems, but I think there are people who draw into themselves and do have problems, unless the assistance that is being offered is more pro- active. It sometimes doesn't reach the people it needs to reach. Beirut was the first time that we and

the United States Government facilities were really subjected to this kind of stuff outside the military. It was the early days. My impression is that now, when things like this happen, State is a lot more pro- active in going after people and saying, "Wait a minute, wait a minute, sit down and let's talk."

Gregory said that "when the psychiatrist came, we were supposed to have been informed, but they never told Communications about it. They forgot completely about us."

U.S. civilian employees were granted a special two-week period of R&R in the U.S under a provision of the Foreign Service Act of 1980. Most found the R&R useful. A few did not. One claimed not to have known about the R&R. One Foreign Service Officer was not entitled to a trip back to the States. She was not pleased. Butler thought that the "R&R was a good thing. I needed to be with my family." Smith noted,

> Mine was the first R&R and it was on May 9th. I stayed one week back here in the States. All the family was eager for details, because they had been hearing little reports. To me that was good therapy, to talk about every little thing, because then you're reliving it that final time.

The Crockers did not see the value of returning to Washington. Christine said that they

> didn't go right away. We kept trying to get out of it. We did not want to go to Washington, because it would not have been useful. But they were giving tickets to Washington. We went for a day, and then we went to Ireland. It was the right place to go.

Because of her TDY status, Gregory was told she was not allowed R&R. She felt that

> State did nothing, absolutely nothing for me. I really, really resented [it] for years and years. Well, I still resent the Department of State's attitude on that. Because I did have friends there. For two days, I thought Diane

> Dillard had been killed. They gave everyone in the Embassy but me a special R&R back to the States. They said, "Oh, no, you don't get it. You were just here on temporary duty." Well, what did that have to do with it? I have never found out.

Mission management continued business as usual, with the understanding that anyone who wished could leave Beirut without penalty. This policy was maintained. Gregory was sent from Beirut to Abu Dhabi on TDY, and then back to Beirut. In August 1983, when the city was being shelled, Gregory remembered after her second TDY, Mr. Pugh asked me if I wanted to leave and I said, "I would love to. I don't want to die for Lebanon, I'll tell you." I said, "But I can't. I'm a Rover and I can't just pick up and leave." And he said, "I promise you it won't hurt your career." I went out by helicopter with Carol Madison [a USIS colleague].

Pascoe spoke of the senior management's ability to remain calm and demonstrate leadership.

> I thought Bob Pugh did marvelously in being cool. The security person, Dick Gannon, was very cool and calm and that helps a lot. Diane Dillard went about her business setting up her household, and what more could the department do? I think that they are very good in a crisis to try to help us.

Washington sent in Under Secretary for Political Affairs Lawrence Eagleburger to accompany the coffins back to the States. Later, Secretary of State George Shultz flew to Beirut and met with mission staff. FSOs who mentioned these top-level visits considered them politically correct. However, the extra work that such high-ranking officials imposed upon the staff was not universally appreciated. Christine Crocker mentioned that Washington "sent out their little cast of characters. All it did was create more work. But it was the right thing, and Washington had to do it." Butler thought that,

> Secretary Shultz's visit was both for political reasons to make a statement and for the morale of the people in the Embassy. Frankly, I felt resentful, because we had to go into high gear to tend to his security needs.

> Everybody had to write briefing papers. They had to clear the whole area. Security people had to get to tops of buildings. People had to put themselves at risk in order to allow Shultz to fly in and look at the Embassy. He talked very briefly to staff. He's such an understated person, not an emotive person, that it wasn't particularly an emotional experience to be comforted by him.

Most said that they thought the State Department provided sufficient support, but several had specific suggestions for handling future crises. Shafer believed that "[i]f I were in another embassy that blew up, I would do just exactly what was done in Beirut: take care of physical needs, and then spiritual needs, if you will." According to Dillon, "[t]he personnel people at the Department of State reacted very quickly. Everybody wanted to be helpful." However, Mandel was concerned that his children are still upset about the bombing.

> The biggest problem was notification. They were all in boarding school. I think they still have vivid recollections and a lot of anger about it. There isn't much you can do, but I think that there's got to be a better way.

Lee believed that the State Department

> "could have followed through on me a little bit more, even though I wasn't injured...They didn't talk to everybody that was involved in this bombing. No one contacted me." Gregory felt a bit neglected. "...[T]wo of us worked twelve-hour shifts. I never even got a thank you or a job well done. I got nothing out of that."

For Samuel, losing contact with her colleagues was an issue.

> They never did have a gathering of people. I don't know if they felt that most people just wanted to get on with their lives and forget it, or what. But I think it would have been good for people to get together. I would like to see how people are. People we never saw again.

Several expressed disappointment that the Department of State did not have a ceremony on the tenth anniversary of the bombing of the Beirut Embassy. Pech had asked the Lebanon Desk Officer about a gathering, only to find out that nothing was planned. She was distressed that the CIA had a get-together but had not been in touch with the other agencies. Lee has noticed that "[r]arely, rarely do they mention the bombing of the Embassy...I feel that the Embassy has been pushed in the corner." Samuel was bothered because

> nobody seems to remember that we were bombed first. I mean, there's been no publicity. You never see that date mentioned. I mean, this year nobody mentioned it. The date that everyone talks about is the day the Marines were bombed.

Mandel found,

> ...it was kind of interesting with the ten-year anniversary they held that memorial service for the Marines. I said, "Gee, fine. Think about it for the Marines, but nobody thought about it for all those people that died in the Embassy." At least, I never saw anything like a memorial service like they did for the Marines. It really is funny how the whole institutional memory seems to suppress that, the whole remembrance of it. I think it's part of the cycle of, "Oh God, look what happened. We've got to spend money, spend money." Now all of a sudden we're starting to get this, "Boy, why are we spending all this money on security? Look at this waste of money." We're on a downswing and have been for several years, with budget cuts and deficits. How do we justify this and that?

B.   QUESTIONNAIRE COMPLETED BY FSOs

An anonymous questionnaire was sent to twenty-seven FSOs assigned to Beirut in 1983; fourteen FSOs with whom I had spoken, thirteen with whom I had not. Out of the twenty-seven sent, nineteen (70%) were returned completed.

Of the nineteen FSOs, fifteen (79%) had been with State, three (16%) with AID, and one (5%) with USIS in 1983. Thirteen (68%) were men and six (32%) were women. Eleven (58%) still were working for the government. The remaining eight (42%) had retired.

Preparation for Beirut Assignment

Fifteen (79%) had attended "Coping with Violence Abroad," a one-day workshop conducted by the Foreign Service Institute to prepare staff for overseas living. Two (11%) had had military experience, and three (16%) had served in hardship posts prior to Beirut.

The FSOs were asked what type of pre-departure preparation would be helpful for future Foreign Service Officers. Several had suggestions: confront the reality of terrorism by having FSOs role-play previous terrorist events, by hearing from people who had been involved in terrorist acts, by showing "Crisis Work, Crisis Worker," by giving special post-specific briefings for those assigned to danger posts, and by stressing that one is responsible for knowing about the environment in which one is working.

Reaction to Bombing

The questionnaire listed the thirteen most common reactions to traumatic experiences which include: re-experiencing, avoiding, and arousal reactions. The respondents were asked to note their reactions to the bombing divided by time frames of the first three months following the bombing, three months to ten years later, and now. They could check YES or NO indicating if they had had a similar response. A few times, people who regularly checked each column left a blank. I recorded their "blanks" as NA (not answered). The completed questionnaire is in the Appendix.

For most, the bombing of the Embassy was a psychologically distressing event. Each FSO responded differently. Seventeen (89%) had symptoms of re-experiencing the traumatic event, increased arousal, and, to a limited degree, avoidance of stimuli associated with the bombing.

Two (11%) of the nineteen respondents marked on the questionnaire that they did not have any reaction to the bombing. One claimed never to have had any reactions. The other, however, checked "feeling of detachment about the bombing" and "feeling of detachment toward people" later in the questionnaire, claiming that those feelings began three months after the bombing and continue up to now.

Within the first three months, seventeen (89%) checked symptoms of being "overly vigilant about your surroundings" (fourteen times), "overly jumpy" (eleven times), "unwanted recollections of the bombing" (eight times), and "negative reactions to events, people or places that remind you of the bombing" (six times). The remaining symptoms were selected from one to five times apiece.

From three months to ten years later, seventeen (89%) FSOs continued to have some reactions. Two categories ("unwanted recollections of the bombing" and "feeling you were reliving the bombing") increased. All the other categories either remained the same or were reduced during this time frame.

Fourteen (74%) have reactions up to the present. The remaining five (26%) no longer have any reactions to the bombing. Of the fourteen who still have reactions, ten (71%) have one or two reactions and four (29%) have between four to six reactions. The most frequently cited response (seven times) was "negative reactions to events, people, or places that remind you of the bombing." The two second most common ones, each cited six times, were "unwanted recollections of the bombing" and "overly jumpy." Being "overly vigilant about your surroundings" was marked four times while "dreams or nightmares about the bombing" and "feeling of detachment toward people" were each checked three times. The rest were specified only once or twice.

Only one (5%) FSO cited a sufficient number of stress reactions to suggest possible PTSD.

Follow-up Activities After the Bombing

All but one FSO knew that the State Department had sent two psychiatrists to Lebanon following the explosion. Seven (37%) did not meet with either doctor. Twelve (63%) met with one of the two. Of those twelve, eight (67%) felt that the psychiatrist was not experienced in dealing with people who had been bombed.

When asked with whom they processed their reactions to the bombing, thirteen (68%) cited "family," twelve (63%) marked "friends," four (21%) checked "State Department's Medical Staff" and twelve (63%) indicated "by myself." Only one (5%) marked "private counselor."

Twelve (63%) took an R&R following the bombing. Seven (37%) did not. Reasons given for not taking the R&R included "not authorized" (due to departure from post soon or because of TDY status), "not known it was offered," and "no time." Of those who did return to Washington for a brief visit, six (50%) considered it "essential," four (33%) "helpful," and one (8%) "unnecessary." One simply noted that the R&R was offered too soon after the event.

When asked if they had seen any of the several videos on the processing of trauma made by the State Department, only two (11%) answered affirmatively. The same two had seen all five of the tapes listed. A third person was not sure if he or she had seen "Crisis Work, Crisis Worker." Fourteen (74%) of the FSOs would be willing to talk about their experiences on tape or with FSOs going to danger posts.

Six (32%) noted that someone from their agency had officially asked about their reactions to the bombing. The inquirers included the regional medical officer from Cairo, a psychiatrist sent to Beirut by the State Department's Medical Division, security investigators, the Director of European Affairs, and the producer-writer of the videos on processing trauma and grief.

Ten (53%) FSOs initiated discussion of their experiences of the bombing with their colleagues. Nine (47%) did not.

Four (21%) FSOs have gotten together with their colleagues a few months or years after the bombing to discuss the impact that the bombing had had on their lives. Ten (52%) believed that a gathering of all those in the bombing would perhaps be useful. Nine (47%) did not see the need.

Some FSOs wrote out suggestions for improving the processing of their experience. Their suggestions included: debriefing by the State Department, taping FSOs' experiences immediately after an incident (and making them public), sending psychiatrists experienced in dealing with bombing incidents, holding responsible personnel accountable for the lack of security, being recognized (by AID) for work, dealing with guilt feelings, reassigning FSOs immediately, showing a bit more compassion (State Department), and having a follow-up session with colleagues a year later.

C.   SUMMARY OF FINDINGS

This chapter describes the impact of the bombing of the American Embassy on the FSOs in Beirut. Two sets of data were used, one from an interview and one from a questionnaire.

The bombing of the U.S. Embassy in Beirut in 1983 was a crisis event in that it was a sudden, powerful event outside the range of ordinary experience.

Most of the FSOs in the Embassy at the time of the explosion had a series of emotional reactions symptomatic of post-traumatic stress disorder; however, only one respondent to the questionnaire had a sufficient number of symptoms to suggest chronic post-traumatic stress disorder. One respondent had no reaction to the bombing. The remaining seventeen respondents dealt with one or more stress reactions. Fourteen (74%) experience stress reactions up to the present.

Several possibilities surfaced for the limited number of sustained stress reactions: FSOs were not seriously wounded; FSOs did not have family or close, personal friends killed; FSOs had previous experience of violence in Beirut or other postings; and the competent handling of the situation by top mission management. (Other intuitive explanations, such as that only individuals with strong coping skills select the Foreign Service, or that Foreign Service Officers do experience stress reactions but are unwilling to discuss them, were not mentioned.)

Top mission management focused on work immediately after the bombing. The Deputy Chief of Mission (DCM) held the first of a series of meetings to brief the staff in his apartment several hours after the bombing. Many FSOs said they wanted to work and to be helpful. Several overworked to the point of exhaustion. Some said that they could not relax until after they left Beirut.

Ritual ceremonies were limited: the raising of the American flag over the Embassy the morning after the bombing, the presentation of the caskets at the Beirut airport, the memorial ceremony conducted at the American University of Beirut chapel, and the funeral mass held at Diane Dillard's apartment. Although the events were not numerous, several FSOs mentioned them as being significant, cathartic moments for them.

The State Department's failure to hold a tenth anniversary ceremony of the bombing in 1993 upset several FSOs, who interpreted the lack of recognition as a form of institutional denial that a major tragedy had occurred.

FSOs found certain individual techniques helpful in coping with the bombing. They included: being with the colleagues who experienced the bombing; talking about the incident with family (especially spouses who were with them in Beirut) and Beirut colleagues; putting their emotions on hold and focusing on work; learning about normal stress reactions (and discovering that their reactions were normal); and returning to Beirut following their R&R or after their next assignments.

Although many FSOs spoke about extensive "talk sessions" with family and Beirut colleagues, some FSOs felt constrained in talking about the bombing in depth, especially with their non-Beirut colleagues.

The bombing had a long-term impact on the lives of some FSOs. Some felt "stronger" after the bombing because they knew that they could handle trauma. Others gained an awareness of their own vulnerability and a greater appreciation of life. Several have become acutely aware of security issues.

The State Department provided on-scene support by sending three regional medical doctors (two of whom were psychiatrists) to Beirut following the bombing, authorizing reassignment to anyone wishing to leave Beirut and offering an extraordinary R&R, and having the Deputy Under Secretary for Political Affairs and the Secretary of State visit Beirut.

The meetings with the psychiatrists got a mixed review. Several people interviewed rated some meetings as quite good, others as a waste of time. Several interviewees stated that they did not need a psychiatrist, and one indicated lack of trust of psychiatrists associated with the State Department. About two-thirds of respondents to the questionnaire who met with a psychiatrist did not believe that the doctor had any experience in dealing with victims of terrorism. However, a few FSOs expressed a desire for greater psychological counseling and a debriefing to process the trauma.

Most FSOs considered the R&R useful. Among those who completed the questionnaire, fifty percent of those who took an R&R found it to be "essential."

The visits of the high level officials from Washington were viewed as a political necessity which simply caused extra work for an already exhausted staff.

For most, "Coping with Violence Abroad," the one-day pre-departure seminar in Washington, D.C., was all the preparation the FSOs had. However, a few had military experience, and several had served in other danger posts. Some FSOs suggested that the training section on terrorism be expanded to include role-playing, talks by those who had been victims, viewing "Crisis Work, Crisis Worker," and special post-specific briefing for those assigned to danger posts.

FSOs made suggestions for follow-up activities, which included: group debriefings after a bombing, a follow-up meeting with colleagues a year after an incident, training the medical staff to handle trauma victims, and making tapes of FSOs talking about their experiences immediately after an incident.

The Department of State produced several training videos on processing trauma and grief in the late 1980s, but very few FSOs have seen them.

Some FSOs expressed anger toward the State Department because their families were not notified in a timely fashion, because TDYers were not authorized R&R, and because no one was held accountable for the lack of proper security and the Department distanced itself from the Beirut bombing.

CHAPTER 5

INSTITUTIONAL PROCEDURES AND REACTIONS

Since the bombing in 1983, the State Department has changed the Foreign Service Institute training courses and, in some cases, how FSOs are handled following a traumatic incident.

<u>State Department Procedures in 1983</u>

In 1983 the Foreign Service Institute offered FSOs getting ready to go to post a one- day training program, "Coping with Violence Abroad." The films and lectures dealt with home and office security, travel precautions, and fire safety. There was no in-depth discussion of terrorism or reactions which FSOs might experience following a terrorist attack.

After the 1983 bombing, the Medical Office sent three Regional medical officers, two of whom were psychiatrists,[36] to Beirut. Two arrived directly after the bombing. The third, Dr. Christine Bieniek[37], a psychiatrist who had joined the Foreign Service in 1980, arrived the second week after the bombing. With no set policy or procedure to follow, she spent a week talking individually with FSOs. She also set up group meetings, which were attended by more women than men, mainly the wives of the FSOs. In addition, she met with any Lebanese staff who wished to see her. Dr. Bieniek believed that arriving the second week was good, because during the first week the FSOs were "dealing with the nitty gritty [of the bombing] and had their feelings on hold." To demonstrate how some FSOs were still in denial, she gave the example of how one person became upset when talking about the plumbing in the apartment building, but remained calm and flat during a discussion of the bombing.

Dr. Bieniek recalled that there were two issues which trouble the FSOs and their spouses: some FSOs were worried about curtailing their tour, in spite of the Ambassador's assurance that their transfers would not penalize their careers (one FSO was concerned about how the promotion board would view his departure), and some wives were upset over the discussion of the possible removal of spouses.

When asked why the Medical Officer had no formal follow-up program, Dr. Bieniek explained that it is the Ambassador who invites psychiatrists to the mission, not the Medical Office, and that regional psychiatrists already have heavy schedules.

The State Department authorized a two-week R&R in Washington for permanent staff after the bombing.

Inman Report in 1985

An Advisory Panel on Overseas Security, chaired by Bobby R. Inman, submitted its report[38] (known as the Inman Report) to the Secretary of State in June 1985. The Inman Report was significant because it provided the basis for a budget and the operational restructuring of security activities. The Panel recommended that the operational security activities be consolidated into a new Bureau for Diplomatic Security (DS) within the State Department and that AID and USIS security programs be consolidated with those of DS[39]. The Panel also recommended improvements in the physical security standards overseas.

The Panel made several recommendations which directly affected the training and handling of FSOs involved in terrorist acts. The Panel recommended improving the missions' contingency plans, specifically citing the expansion of the crisis management simulation exercise program; improving the training of FSOs and their dependents to deal more effectively with terrorism and other forms of violence overseas; providing adequate levels of psychological preparation for overseas situations; lengthening "Coping with Violence Abroad" to include the psychological aspects of terrorist incidents; and ensuring that all FSOs attend the training. The Panel also acknowledged that even though the Office of the Medical Adviser was understaffed, it was able to play a major role in preparing the FSOs for coping with terrorist violence.[40]

Congress passed the "Omnibus Diplomatic Security and Antiterrorism Act of 1986" to enhance diplomatic security and to combat international terrorism. A new Bureau of Diplomatic Security of the Department of State, headed by an Assistant Secretary of State, was created. With the support of the Secretary of State, Congress allotted money to improve the security of U.S. embassies, to prepare FSOs for danger posts, and to increase the psychiatric staff of the Medical Office.

State Department Procedures in 1994

The Overseas Briefing Center of the Foreign Service Institute, Department of State, replaced "Coping with Violence Abroad" with "Security Overseas Seminar" (SOS) in 1988, five years after the Beirut bombing. The updated two-day course covers a variety of security issues, ranging from "What To Do About Bombs" to "Managing in a Crisis." New FSOs and their families are scheduled to attend the seminar prior to going abroad. In addition, FSOs are required now to attend SOS every five years. Personnel officers are charged with the responsibility of insuring that FSOs posted abroad attend SOS when back in Washington on leave. According to DanaDee Carragher[41], Coordinator for SOS, forty-seven percent of the FSOs who attend SOS have taken the course previously, but she does not have a record of how many FSOs actually sign up every five years.

The last lecture of the second day of SOS is given by a mental health specialist, who has an hour and fifteen minutes to review the symptoms frequently experienced following trauma. Due to time constraints, FSOs have an opportunity to mention, but not discuss in detail, their personal experiences. Cay Hartley[42], a clinical social worker who frequently gives this lecture, said that about two-thirds of her audiences have had traumatic experiences.

Not all of the FSOs stay for the entire two days of SOS. Carragher says that about ten percent of the participants leave directly after lunch on the second day and, therefore, do not hear the lecture on stress management.

Among the materials given to the participants are "Action Strategies" and "SOS Handbook." Both have sections on recognizing and managing stress. "Foreign Service Assignment Notebook"[43] has a chapter on the stress of cultural shock, but does not deal with trauma associated with natural disaster or terrorism.

A variety of videos, including those concerned with stress and grief, are available, but not shown as part of the training session.

A test pilot of a one-day Advanced SOS is being offered to those who have attended SOS previously. It will be incorporated into the fall schedule of 1994.

The Foreign Service Institute also gives special seminars[44] for Ambassadors and Deputy Chiefs of Mission, but the courses do not include a lecture on the psychological effects of trauma.

The State Department Mental Health Services now has ten regional psychiatrists and two psychiatrists in Washington. In 1980, Dr. Esther P. Roberts[45], Associate Medical Director of Mental Health Services, helped set up the office which she now directs. Not long after its establishment, she was designing a Protocol for the FSOs held hostage by Iran. She debriefed the FSOs upon their release and also followed up with them six months later. She is still in contact with some of them and their families. Dr. Roberts mentioned that one impediment her office faces today is inadequate feedback on the FSOs and their families. There is no follow-up because the institution (personnel) does not require it.

Dr. Roberts noted that critical incident stress debriefings were given to FSOs from Kuwait and Iraq during the Gulf war, but they are not a routine procedure. Some mental health workers support doing routine debriefings for FSOs whenever a catastrophic crisis occurs. Hartley advocates group debriefing, because the setting allows all present to get the same information, hear about the stress reactions of others, and learn that their reactions are normal. Repetition of stress management techniques is needed, she added, because during trauma the brain gets "scrambled," and one forgets what one knows.

The State Department does not have a uniform procedure for handling FSOs involved in terrorism. The reason, Dr. Roberts believes, is that each incident is different, depending on the nature of the crisis. She laughingly suggested that "wishful denial" may be a component.

Diplomatic Security (DS) became a Bureau as a result of the Inman Report. DS expanded its educational functions to include conducting simulations of crisis training and making videos on the human side of crisis management. The videos were made in conjunction with The Overseas Briefing Center, the Medical Division, Family Liaison Office, and Consular Affairs. The tapes are sent to the Regional Security Officer and the Community Liaison Office at post.

In making videos on stress management, DS has used Elmore F. Rigamer, a psychiatrist who is presently the Medical Director of the Department of State, and Sheila Platt, a clinical social worker who is presently doing critical incident stress debriefing for the United Nations staff in the Balkans. Platt, as the wife of an Ambassador serving in several critical posts, has had first-hand exposure in overseas political and natural disaster trauma. She has applied Jeffrey Mitchell's theory that disaster workers are "hidden" victims of a disaster to FSOs involved in traumatic events. Platt[46] makes an analogy between Mitchell's "hidden" victims, those who help survivors, and FSOs. "Foreign Service Officers who don't have training themselves do not think of themselves as disaster workers," she said.

Accepting the reality of being in disaster is a

> ...new concept for Foreign Service people. They had no sort of permission to be affected by any of this stuff. Even professional mental health people tend to think training and experience protect them from reacting. Forget it. Of course, they are going to react, but they may be better equipped to handle their reactions or know where to go to get assistance if needed.

Platt believes firmly in educating FSOs about stress prior to their encountering a disaster. "What helps people is to know their reaction is normal." She also highly values group debriefing after the disaster. The process, Platt thinks, needs to be "de-shrinked." Using the analogy of a broken leg, Platt explained the person needs to be told about the healing process and not to expect to be riding a bike for a while. Platt says someone needs to say, "Tell me what's happening with you, and we'll talk about what stage you are at..."

The Family Liaison Office and the Association of American Foreign Service Women Evacuee Support Network work directly with FSOs and, especially, their dependents in times of crisis. The Employee Consultation Service, which was started five years ago, offers counseling services to FSOs and their families. (Their records are NOT sent to the State Medical office or their personnel files.)

CHAPTER 6

CONCLUSIONS AND RECOMMENDATIONS

Conclusions

Most FSOs in Beirut had not been prepared for working in a war zone and, when caught up in the bombing, they continued work, "business as usual," without fully acknowledging the traumatic effect the bombing had on their lives. Many FSOs worked to the point of exhaustion and did not relax until they left Lebanon. As a result, they may have delayed the process of healing the psychological wounds caused by the explosion.

FSOs did not pressure the Department to provide additional psychological support, because many either saw no need for it or did not value the concept of psychiatry and/or the competency of some of the psychiatrists working within the Department.

The vast majority of FSOs experienced—and some still do today—a series of post- traumatic stress reactions; however, only one FSO described symptoms which may indicate a full blown post-traumatic stress disorder. Since several were unaware that their reactions were normal in light of the catastrophic event, one can only conclude that FSOs were not educated in the psychological ramifications of trauma. Although most FSOs instinctively worked through their emotional reactions by talking to colleagues and family, all may not have processed fully their reactions to the bombing. Some may not have acknowledged the need to recognize and process the trauma of the bombing.

After the bombing, FSOs wanted to help each other. They exhibited a "we can handle what ever happens" attitude and a sense of loyalty toward their Beirut colleagues. Several stressed that, in spite of the bombing, they still enjoyed being in the Foreign Service.

Top mission management in Beirut fully supported the FSOs after the bombing by requesting regional psychiatrists, authorizing an extraordinary R&R, and offering the option of immediate reassignments. Although it was not a guided group critical incident stress debriefing (CISD) as developed by Jeffrey Mitchell, the DCM's daily meeting seemed to function as one, to the degree that the FSOs had an opportunity to share their reactions and anxieties with one another.

The Department of State does not yet officially acknowledge that violence has a long-term effect on those involved, even if only indirectly involved. If they had, education about the effects of trauma would have been built into the existing training programs at *all* levels and relevant staff would have been trained to handle FSOs confronting trauma. By not paying attention to the FSOs' experience in Beirut, the State Department's indifference, a form of institutional denial, camouflaged the significance of their trauma. The predominant Foreign Service culture has yet to rid itself of the outdated attitude that any attention to mental health betrays a weakness. The notion that using the services of educators and counselors as a form of preventive medicine and a way of educating oneself on normal human development has not caught hold.

Not all of the FSOs, including the Ambassadors and the Deputy Chiefs of Mission, receive the psychological preparation and follow-up necessary for today's Foreign Service. The State Department has tended to compartmentalize the responsibilities for the education of and support of FSOs. Individual offices have made a contribution toward educating FSOs on post-traumatic stress, but the efforts are not integrated within a system.

Although cognizant that Beirut was a danger post, most FSOs were not prepared for the reality of the bombing. The Department of State seminar, "Coping with Violence Abroad," was not sufficient preparation. Even though the subsequent "Security Overseas Seminar" (SOS), and various training videos on the psychological aspects of trauma and stress management were developed (after the Beirut bombing), not all FSOs benefit from them because of a lack of administrative tracking. No foolproof method of scheduling FSOs for SOS every five years, or of showing the training videos overseas, exists. Currently, due to budgetary cutbacks, Diplomatic Security's crisis management simulation exercise program and its videomaking capacity have been eliminated.

Information on the psychological impact of terrorism is not "linked" to the Ambassadors, who are responsible for the FSOs overseas. During the week-long training sessions for top management, the Foreign Service Institute no longer briefs all Ambassadors and DCMs on the predictable reactions of trauma, and the need to facilitate recovery by processing feelings following trauma. Nor are the videotapes dealing with these issues sent to the Ambassadors in the missions. (They are sent to the RSO/CLO.)

The Medical Office does not have a standard policy or a protocol for handling and following up on FSOs who have encountered terrorism, but rather reacts to each political situation on a case by case basis. The State Department had its medical staff conduct critical incident stress debriefings for officers involved in highly publicized political events, such as the Iran hostage situation and the Gulf War, but does not carry out group debriefings or CISDs as a matter of routine procedure for less publicized events. Crisis management may well be necessary in the political arena; however, procedures for handling FSOs who survive trauma should be standardized. In addition, the quality of care of FSOs should be the same for both low- and high-profile situations.

No office has the responsibility of ensuring that Ambassadors and medical staff are trained in dealing with victims of terrorism.

Recommendations

Develop a policy based on the recognition that stress (and often catastrophic stress) caused by international terrorism and political turmoil has become a norm for Foreign Service Officers; openly provide crisis intervention and follow-up to those FSO involved in overseas trauma.

Educate all those in the Foreign Service about post-traumatic stress and how to manage it. Insure that Ambassadors and DCMs, especially political appointees who have not had the benefit of hardship posts or military experience, are informed about the psychological aspects of terrorism. At a minimum, top management should be given the same information which is presented to Foreign Service Officers in the "Security Overseas Seminar."

Train members of the health care units at the missions, as well as the regional psychiatrists, in critical incident stress debriefing techniques. Contract U.S. and, if available, local mental health workers to support Foreign Service Officers following a disaster.

APPENDICES

APPENDIX A

LIST OF INTERVIEWEES

Tish Butler

Christine Crocker

Ryan Crocker

Diane Dillard

Robert Dillon

Dick Gannon

Barbara Gregory

Faith Lee

David H. Mandel

Dorothy Pascoe

Dorothy Pech

Daniel J. Pellegrino*

Beth Samuel

Kurt Shafer

Rebecca Smith

* Member of the defense attaché's office who was interviewed. His remarks were not incorporated with the others'. However, an edited version of his interview is in the appendix along with those of the Foreign Service Officers.

APPENDIX B

INTERVIEW – OPEN-ENDED QUESTIONS (11/93)

I would like to ask you about three things:

1. Your reaction to the Beirut bombing:
   How it affected you in 1983 and if it affects you today.
2. Your assessment as to why it happened.
3. Your suggestions for helping FSOs deal with traumatic episodes such as terrorist activities or natural disasters.

Would it be all right if I tape our conversation so I don't have to worry about missing anything you have to say?

May I use your name or do you want me not to identify you?

1. Background questions:

Name: Agency:

Address: (in 1983)

Phone:

How long had you been a FSO: # of tours in Middle East:

Why did you go to Beirut?

Did you leave the Mideast because of the bombing:

Did you have any previous traumatic experience:

Why do you think the Embassy was bombed? How did it happen?

2. Bombing

Where were you at the time of the bombing? What happened to you?

How do you feel about the bombing today?

3. Follow-up

What was done to help you and your colleagues to deal with the stress? (Who provided it? Was it practical/sufficient?

What else could have been done?)

        4.   Integration

What kind of sense do you make of it? (How do you see that the bombing has made a difference in your life? Changed your life? How you view work?)

        5.   Suggestions

How prepared were you for this terrorist trauma?

What suggestions do you have for preparing and following up on FSOs who are sent to danger posts and/or become victims of terrorism?

        6.   Impact - first year(s)

How did the bombing affect you at first? During the first few months, years? (Stress reactions: nightmares, etc.)

Comfortable discussing your reactions with colleagues, friends?

At the end of January, I plan to send out an anonymous, YES-NO questionnaire to the FSOs who were in the Embassy. I would appreciate your completing it, even though you have already touched upon some of the points today.

APPENDIX C

FOREIGN SERVICE OFFICERS WHO WERE SENT QUESTIONNAIRE (27)

Tom Barron	David Mandel
Tish Butler	Dundas McCullough
Christine Crocker	Catherine Nylund
Ryan Crocker	Don Nylund
Philo Dibble	Dorothy Pascoe
Diane Dillard	Dorothy Pech
Robert Dillon	Lisa Piascik
Robert Essington	Robert Pugh
Dennis Foster	John Reid
Dick Gannon	Beth Samuel
Barbara Gregory	Kurt Shafer
Hunt Janin	Paul Siekert
Bill Lamb	Rebecca O. Smith
Faith Lee	

APPENDIX D

QUESTIONNAIRE

On April 18, 1983, at 1:05 p.m. a truck weighted down with over 2,000 pounds of TNT drove into the front door of the U.S. Embassy in Beirut.

In the fall of 1993, for a master's degree thesis from Georgetown University, I started my preliminary literature research on the political ramifications of that bombing. Very little has been written on the bombing. Only a few articles (and no books) detail an event that altered not only our foreign policy, but also the way in the which our embassies and staff are protected. I began to wonder why so little has been written about the Embassy. I thought about my colleagues who had died. I also thought about my colleagues who had lived. What were their thoughts on the tenth anniversary of the bombing? How did the explosion affect their lives? How did they handle the injury and death that had surrounded them? Could their experience be of help to the men and women living in danger posts today? To answer these questions, I began interviewing those colleagues whom I could reach by phone.

To widen the circle to include all who worked for AID, State, and USIS, I am sending out this anonymous questionnaire with the hopes of gaining your insight and experience. I would appreciate hearing from you. Thank you for taking the time to complete the form and returning it to me in the enclosed, stamped envelope.

Please check the appropriate spaces:

19 responses: Male 13 Female 6 Working 11 Retired 8 While in Beirut, for whom did you work?

3 AID; 15 State; 1 USIS

1. PRE-BEIRUT

Did you attend the Foreign Service Institute Workshop "Coping with Violence Abroad"?

    15 YES   4 NO

Did you have any other training to prepare you for a danger post?

    5 YES   14 NO

If yes, list: Hardship posts (2); military (2); seminars (1)

2. BOMBING

Were you in the Embassy when it was bombed?

    17 YES   2 NO

If not, where were you? Home (1); Sidon, Lebanon (1)

People have varying reactions to traumatic experiences. Some of the most common ones are listed below. Some people react shortly after the traumatic event; others have a delayed reaction.

Question	1st 3 mos.	3 mos-10 yrs	To present
Did you have a reaction to the bombing?	Yes 17 No 2 NA 0	Yes 17 No 2 NA 0	Yes 14 No 5 NA 0

If yes, please note your reactions:

unwanted recollections of the bombing	Yes 8 No 11 NA 0	Yes 9 No 10 NA 0	Yes 6 No 12 NA 1
dreams or nightmares about the bombing	Yes 4 No 15 NA 0	Yes 5 No 13 NA 1	Yes 3 No 16 NA 0
feeling you were reliving the bombing	Yes 5 No 14 NA 0	Yes 6 No 13 NA 0	Yes 2 No 16 NA 1
negative reactions to events, people or places that remind you of the bombing	Yes 6 No 12 NA 1	Yes 9 No 9 NA 1	Yes 7 No 10 NA 2
trouble remembering parts of the bombing	Yes 2 No 17 NA 0	Yes 3 No 16 NA 0	Yes 2 No 17 NA 0

loss of interest in hobbies or special interests	Yes 2 No 16 NA 1	Yes 1 No 18 NA 0	Yes 1 No 18 NA 0
feeling of detachment about the bombing	Yes 3 No 16	Yes 2 No 17	Yes 2 No 17
feeling of detachment toward people	Yes 2 No 17	Yes 2 No 17	Yes 3 No 16

Question	1st 3 mos.	3 mos-10 yrs	To present
difficulty sleeping	Yes 5 No 14	Yes 4 No 15	Yes 1 No 18
increase in irritability	Yes 3 No 16	Yes 2 No 17	Yes 1 No 18
difficulty concentrating	Yes 4 No 15	Yes 4 No 15	Yes 1 No 18
overly vigilant about your surroundings	Yes 14 No 5	Yes 10 No 9	Yes 4 No 15
overly jumpy	Yes 11 No 8	Yes 9 No 10	Yes 6 No 13
cried a lot [added by responder]	Yes 1	Yes 1	

3. POST BOMBING

Did you know that the State Department sent out two psychiatrists (a man and a woman) following the bombing?

    18 YES   1 NO

Did you meet with either one?

    12 YES   6 NO 1 NA

If yes, did you feel the psychiatrist was experienced in dealing with those who had undergone a bombing?

    3 YES   8 NO 1 NA

With whom did you process your reactions to the bombing? (Check one or more.)

    13 family   12 friends
  4 State Med staff 1 private counselor 12 by myself

Did you take the R&R offered after the bombing?

     12 YES   7 NO

If no, why not? 2 Not know offered 1 On TDY 3 No time

    1 Had only two months left at post.

If yes, did you find it:

    1 unnecessary 4 helpful 6 essential

    1 offered too soon after the event

Do you know that since 1986 the State Department has made several videos on processing trauma?

     2 YES   15 NO

Have you had the opportunity to see:

1. Crisis Work, Crisis Worker	3 YES	14 NO	2 NA
2. Grief Cycle: Notification of Death	2 YES	16 NO	1 NA
3. Managing A Crisis: Before, During and After	2 YES	16 NO	1 NA
4. Crisis Abroad: An Embassy Responds	2 YES	16 NO	1 NA
5. They Shall Not Have Died in Vain	2 YES	16 NO	1 NA

Did anyone from your agency ever officially ask you about your reactions to the bombing?

     6 YES   13 NO

If yes, from which office? 2 DS 1 Cairo doctor-

1 State psychiatrist 1 Security investigator

1 Director of European Affairs

Did you initiate discussion of your experience with your colleagues?

     10 YES   9 NO

Today, would you be willing to talk about your experience on tape or with FSOs going to danger posts?

     15 YES   2 NO 2 PERHAPS

Have you ever gotten together with all your colleagues a few months/years after the bombing to discuss the impact that it has had on your lives?

     4 YES   15 NO

[If no,] would such a meeting have been useful?

1 NA   8 YES   7 NO   3 PERHAPS

LOOKING BACK AT YOUR EXPERIENCE, WHAT WOULD HAVE BEEN HELPFUL TO YOU IN PROCESSING YOUR EXPERIENCE OF THE BOMBING?

1. DEBRIEFING:

    A. Probably a debriefing when I finally departed Beirut.

    B. The State Department oral history program could have been used to record the experiences of many of those involved, particularly while the experience was quite fresh in everyone's mind.

2. PSYCHIATRISTS:

    I believe I should, in fact, have met with the... psychiatrists. Talking to family and friends is important, but professional input as to why we react as we do, and what possibly to expect, might have made later experiences less frightening.

3. ACCOUNTABILITY:

    A. Not giving awards, as was done, to those who contributed to the extent of the disaster (e.g., lax security) for what they did to clean up the mess.

    B. Having those in the Embassy held accountable for their lack of concern prior to the bombing, and relieving those who were uncaring/ineffective in running the mission.

4. RECOGNITION:

    Recognition by AID for the efforts we all made after the bombing to get back to work and keep the program going.

5. DANGER PAY:

    The State Department should have given danger pay to all of us right after the bombing. Only the Marines got it—before and after. The Department finally gave it, some of it retroactively, a year or so after I left Beirut in July '83. The Department consistently tried to downplay medical injuries I incurred before and during the bombing.

6. GUILT:

To shed all feelings of guilt—the gift that keeps on giving. I'll never forget a visitor from another agency who met me at Khalil's in Animerisi and blamed me for all the deaths, [the] maimed and the para/quadraplegics. He was young and angry and, while I didn't like it, I knew he spoke from ignorance. His colleagues dragged him away while "explaining" that no one had done more to prevent just such a bombing. The odd thing is, I felt I should have done even more to get Washington to react faster to my recommendations. So—I felt, and still feel guilt, but he was the only one to give that latent guilt a boost. FYI, the Joint Agency Task Force placed the entire blame on Washington for squabbling amongst themselves and ignoring my pleading for action on "hardening" the Embassy and installing several anti-terrorism devices. I ended up with all kinds of awards, etc., but was in such a depression that I "slept" all night—and day. I'd stop breathing 30-40 times a day and wake up gasping for air. In that condition, I couldn't get a job (although European Affairs gave me an office and I should stay on and work whenever I felt I could, on whatever I wanted to do). So I was given 100% disability discharge. I'm much improved, but still haunted.

LOOKING TOWARD THE FUTURE, WHAT TYPE OF PREPARATION AND FOLLOW-UP DO YOU THINK WOULD BE HELPFUL FOR FOREIGN SERVICE OFFICERS INVOLVED IN TERRORIST ATTACKS?

1. PREPARATION AND ORIENTATION:

   A. ROLE PLAYING:

   ...confronting the reality of terrorist events, perhaps in role-playing what had actually occurred in several previous terrorist incidents, would, in my view, be helpful as preparation for service in particularly dangerous posts. This might be done as an extension of the "Coping With Violence Abroad" seminar.

   B. TALKS:

   Talks from people who have undergone such experiences. And why not—if possible—talks from reformed terrorists (at least on video or deposition/transcript to understand what motivates them.)

C. VIDEOS:

"Crisis Work, Crisis Worker" and video on grief might be useful. Those new videos sound useful.

D. SPECIAL BRIEFINGS:

Anyone going into a danger post for the first time should have a personal, special briefing—post-specific. In the case of Beirut, it should be designed to scare the daylights out of all personnel. FSOs are sometimes too self-confident in matters of security.

E. SUPPLIES:

Each person, especially secretaries, should be instructed to have an emergency pack at hand. This should include paper, pens, telephone numbers, etc., so that when sent to another site, they can start right up.

F. EMBASSY PRE-PLAN:

It is important for the embassy managers to be prepared, organized, and ready to act. If senior levels have a plan that really works—e.g., not overly complex, involves <u>everyone</u>—the first hour following the event will help rather than hinder recovery from shock and fear.

There should be many more, and more realistic (i.e., unexpected) emergency drills. These should simulate various scenarios, especially breaks in the chain of command due to absence, injury, or death, and ideally should last at least 24 hours.

G. ASSUME RESPONSIBILITY:

Be aware that it can happen to you…Accept responsibility for your own security. Know the environment in which you are working. Ask questions. Take the RSO's briefing seriously. Don't set consistent patterns of movement. If it happens, look for ways to be helpful in coping with the aftermath, even if that is not in your job description. If you're not hurt, don't expect to be taken care of. Look for ways to stay busy that contribute to the general welfare.

H. REASSIGN:

Also, failure of the Department [in the first bombing] to immediately take survivors out and reassign [them] as they did in the second bombing shows complete lack of concern for the well-being of employees.

I. PERSONNEL:

The State Department could show a bit more compassion. I remember one young man that had been badly wounded in the second Beirut bombing approached me as his Personnel Technician, stating he was getting the run-around. He had no idea of where to go in the Department, what to do. Since I had been through it, I had him give me all the things he needed answered and done, and I then called around the building getting answers. He was so appreciative. He had felt no one cared or gave a darn.

2. POST BOMBING:

A. MEDICAL:

The best follow-up is good medical care, delivered quickly,... well-prepared contingency plans for providing it. I'm not a believer in psychological and psychiatric analysis.

[Staff experienced in trauma.] Lack of concern by the visiting psychiatrists also bothers me...all she could ask was, "Well, how do you feel about the death of your friends?"

B. DEBRIEFING:

There should be an intensive debrief[ing] with someone who understands what the person has experienced.

C. FOLLOW-UP:

A follow-up a year later with others who were involved would be useful.

D. R&R:

R&R/trip home was very important to break out of the crisis mentality and start moving forward.

E. TAPE:

...experiences, good or bad, should be taped immediately after an incident and made public.

3. COMMENTS:

A. Faultfinding is sterile and too late to be helpful.

B. INNER PEACE:

1. Most [FSOs affected by terrorism] who survived had to rely on inner peace, meditation, patience, etc., to maintain their existence... but what emotional scars will remain with them FOREVER?...Keep communications open with fellow employees at all times, if possible.

2. How one reacts to a terrorist incident probably is far more a function of the inner resources one has garnered up to that point in life than it is of the formal preparation one might receive in anticipation of a specific assignment. It was quite clear in the hours, days, and weeks following the attack on the Embassy who had those inner resources and who did not.

C. ACCOUNTABILITY:

Failure of the Department to hold anyone accountable for lack of prior planning still bothers me very much.

D. DANGER POSTING:

...FSOs should not be put in places where such attacks are expected, except on a volunteer basis, as was the case in Beirut...

E. ACCEPT TERRORISM AS A NORM:

The principal effect of the bombing on me was that following it, and until today, I get scared more easily than I used to. This is not a great problem, however.

Unfortunately, terrorism is a problem that we have to live with...You have to be able to accept it, along with natural disasters and other hazards of this job, or else look for another job. I guess that's the bottom line.

F. ASSIGNMENTS:

...there is little competition for assignment to a post like Beirut and agencies usually end up assigning whomever is willing to go; and this is unlikely to change.

APPENDIX E

SURVIVING AMERICAN EMPLOYEES IN BEIRUT[47]

STATE EMPLOYEES:

Executive section:
Robert Dillon
Robert Pugh
Dorothy Pascoe
Dorothy Pech

Political section:
Ryan Crocker
Dennis Foster
Bruce Johnson
Catherine Nylund

Political/military:
Donald Ellson

Economic/commercial section:
Hunt Janin
Murray McCann
Christine Crocker

Consular section:
Diane Dillard
Philo Dibble
Lisa Piascik
Dundas McCullough

Administrative section:
Tom Barron
Robert Essington
Paul Siekert

Communications section:
Faith Lee
Raymond Miller
Leo Pezzi
Don Nylund
Don Chubb

Security:
Dick Gannon
William Lamb
Lawrence Liptack

On temporary duty:
Rick Browning
Frederick King
Barbara Gregory
David Roberts
Michael Mosley
Sue Morgan
Andrew Wartell

The Habib mission:
Philip Habib
Morris Draper
Christopher Ross
Andrew Cooley
Michael G. Kozak
Mary Regan
Louise Tennant
David Anthony

USIS EMPLOYEES:
John Reid
Beth Samuel

AID EMPLOYEES:
Rebecca O. Smith
Ronald Kurt Shafer
Letitia Kelly Butler
David H. Mandel
Anne Dammarell
Robert Pearson

DEPARTMENT OF COMMERCE:
Al Alexander

MARINE SECURITY GUARDS:
Clarence Hardeman
Brian K. Korn
John O. Kreter
Charles Allen Light
Luis Garcia Lopez, Jr.
Jacques L. Massengill
Robert S. Moreno
Charles Thomas Pearson
Ronnie Victor Tumolo
Stanley E. Whitfield

DEFENSE ATTACHÉ'S OFFICE:
Winchell M. Craig
Joseph P. Englehardt
Daniel J. Pellegrino
Sally Johnson

MILITARY TRAINING TEAM:
Rayford J. Byers

APPENDIX F

LEBANESE STAFF KNOWN TO HAVE DIED

Riyad Abul-Massih
Abdallah Al-Halabi
Mohamedain Hassan Assaran
Elias Atallah
Cesar Bathiard
Antoine Dakkash
Mounir Dandan
Farouk Fanous
Raja Iskanderani
Nazih Juraydini
Antoine Karam
Edgard Khouri
Hafez Khouri
Amal Maakaroun
Mary Metni
Mohammed Najja
Nabil Rahhal
Roudayna Sahyoun
Fouad Salameh
Shane Setrakian
Souad Srouh

APPENDIX G

MISSING STAFF PRESUMED TO BE DEAD

Yolla Al-Hashim

Rafic Eid

Hussein Haidar-Ahmad

Mohammed Hassan

Mohammad Ibrahim

Ghazi Kabbout

Raymond Karkour

Kamal Nahhas

Dariniche Ra'i

Khalil Yatim

Riad (last name not known)

Shahine (last name not known)

APPENDIX H

INJURED STAFF

Louise Alrassl

Bedros Anserian

Mary Apovian

Clemance Azouri

Fouad Copti

Hafiz Farah

Hikmat Fayez

Samir Jabbour

Nadwa Jamal

Joseph Karam

Elias Khoury

Majdi Saikali

Anjel Shekerjian

Houda Shuweiry

Anl Srabian

Maggie Teen

APPENDIX I

LIST OF THOSE INTERVIEWED

Christine Bieniek, psychiatrist, Department of State

Peter Block, organization management consultant, Designed Learning

DanaDee Carragher, Foreign Service Institute, Department of State

Margaret Clancy, psychiatrist, private practice

Marius Deeb, Department of Political Science, George Washington University

Mary Jane Deeb, School of International Service, American University

Norman Finkle, Department of Psychiatry, Georgetown University

Bonnie Green, Director of Trauma Studies, Georgetown University

Cay Hartley, psychologist, Counseling and Training Resources, Inc.

Marilyn Holmes, Writer/Producer, Department of State

Linda Olesen, Family Liaison Office, Department of State

Sheila Platt, social psychologist, private practice

Esther Roberts, Associate Medical Director of Mental Health Services, Department of State

Rita Siebenaler, Employee Consultation Services, Department of State

Mallory Starr, psychologist, private practice

APPENDIX J

INTERVIEWS

Edited interview Tish Butler
February 14, 1994 Program Officer in 1983

Peter [McPhearson, Administrator of the Agency for International Development], asked Malcolm [my husband] to be Mission Director. Congress had just appropriated $200 million for Lebanon. Malcolm was to expand the program. We were called on a Friday in September and gone by Sunday a week, unable to cancel all our outstanding social engagements. Some thought we were PNGed!

On the day of the bombing, I got back to my office about five past one. I had put my head into Kurt Shafer's office and got some M&Ms from him. I sat at my desk to study French. The desk was in a catty-corner position, no longer directly in front of the french doors, which is where it had been a week earlier. I remember days afterwards, a week afterwards, when I knew what had happened, a sensation of, like, a drop in pressure that preceded the beginning of a very long rolling, booming sound. At the very tail end of the boom, the room shook. I was knocked halfway to the floor. I wasn't knocked completely to the floor, because I caught myself. The glass in the french doors imploded into the room and passed me on my left. My immediate reaction was that there had been a bomb, either outside the back of the building or right outside my window, because my windows had blown in. I remembered the advice that we had received: if there was any disruption outside, don't run to the window. Run in the opposite direction. I jumped up with my heart pounding and went to the door and had to yank it with all my weight a couple of times. I finally yanked it open. I went down the hallway towards the central corridor. To the right I saw a tremendous amount of smoke and dust particles, particularly in that atrium area directly up from the main foyer on the first floor. I turned left and went towards the main offices of AID and encountered several local staff coming out looking very dazed. They weren't injured. They were just looking frightened and dazed. I remember grabbing one young secretary and holding her real firmly trying to calm her hysteria. Somebody led Mary Lee McIntyre out of the Director's bathroom where she had been during the bombing. She took the force of the bathroom window glass in her face. She was being led, because her eyes were closed. Blood was pooled up in her eyes and streaming down her white, white face. With her white hair, it was really an extraordinary scene.

I remember feeling a strong sense of responsibility to try to pull the group together and to decide what to do to make sure everybody was o.k. I was scared, since I didn't know where the bomb had come from and was afraid that some gas stored in the Embassy might explode. I felt the need for us to get out of the building. We moved towards the central staircase and headed down two floors. We were on the fourth floor. Somebody who preceded me went all the way down and saw that we couldn't get out of the front part. We all started to climb out a second-story window leading to the back. A shack had been built up against the building. We crawled out of the window onto the roof of that shack. There was a ladder leaning on the roof of the shack. As we started to go down the ladder, flames came out of the administrative officer's office just below us. We quickly went back up. I guess there had been some sort of gas tank in his office. I can't remember how we got down, but there was a ladder and people were helping us. Joe and Samir, the drivers, were very solicitous. As I got down to the ground, all I could see was the back and west side of the building. I never saw the front of the building. For 24 or 36 hours, I didn't have a clue of what had really happened.

I went directly from the back of the building into an ambulance with Mary Lee. The ambulance was just a metal box with a cot in it. The driver just tore off like a bat out of hell and careened down the street. I was holding her in place on the cot and finally had to wedge my feet against one side of the truck and my body against her, with my hand on the other side of the truck to try and keep my place. A first-tour officer was also in the ambulance. Brand new. He arrived for duty that morning. He was in shock. His eyes were about as round as saucers and he couldn't hear me talking from the back of the ambulance. It seemed to take years to get to American University Hospital. We had to go down to the corniche[48] and wind our way through the Hamra area. The traffic was bad. I thought we would never get there. We pulled in and I helped Mary Lee out. I then walked into the body area of the hospital where the doctors had set up a triage. There were doctors and people with bandages and cuts and stitches and blood and glassy-eyes everywhere. Just about every doctor and nurse on staff was there. Stitches were flying and there was extraordinary busyness on the part of the staff. It looked to me like there were dozens and dozens of wounded people sitting around. I wanted to assure myself you and Bob Pearson were o.k., or that you were being attended to. You could barely whisper. I found Bob on a gurney out in the lobby. The doctor was picking glass out of his forehead. Big, visible pieces of glass. After a little while, they stitched him up. I stood by his side to comfort him. I sort of stroked his leg a little bit so that he knew somebody was there. Finally he had to ask me to stop. Maybe it hurt. Then you were both taken off to be worked on in an inner room, at which point I went off and found Dave and Jill Mandel. The three of us found an administrative room in the hospital that had a telephone with an open international line, and we called Washington to report on the AID people who were hurt. Then the Defense Attaché asked if we would identify bodies in the makeshift morgue in the basement. Jill and I went down. I walked up and down the corridors in the basement towards the door with an impending sense of dread. It was a very strange mixture of revulsion and attraction. Morbid curiosity. I feared that I might not be able to handle it. I

> spent between three and five minutes in the morgue.
> That was the worst part of the whole event for me.

It seared images of bodies and body parts on my consciousness which stuck with me for a while. That was the first time I had ever seen the effects of a powerful force on the human body. There were too many people for the room, and bodies were all over and on the ground. I recognized Fouad the mailroom clerk, whose father was killed twenty years before at the Embassy. He wore a T-shirt that said "target" in French on the front. I saw Janet Stevens, the long-haired journalist, who had been interviewing Bill McIntyre in the cafeteria. She was in a corner with a military guy. He had his hands up and she was almost in a macabre death embrace. That image in particular stuck with me for nights afterwards.

I didn't talk to Malcolm until I got home that night at about six or seven at night. I had misplaced my purse and Abel the driver lent me some money. I remember taking a big tumbler of liquor to go to sleep.

The next day...we were all called to the Deputy Chief of Mission's apartment. Bob Pugh gave us a rundown on what had happened and the damages that we had. The plan was to be "business as usual." We could not allow the bombing to be successful in terms of letting us fall apart or leave. We would be moving our offices into the Duraffourd Apartments. Bob announced that Secretary Shultz would be coming in. Secretary Shultz's visit was both for political reasons to make a statement, and for the morale of the people in the Embassy. Frankly, I felt resentful, because we had to go into high gear to tend to his security needs. Everybody had to write briefing papers. They had to clear the whole area. Security people had to get to tops of buildings. People had to put themselves at risk in order to allow Shultz to fly in and look at the Embassy. He talked very briefly to staff. He's such an understated person, not an emotive person, that it wasn't particularly an emotional experience to be comforted by him.

Two weeks or a month afterwards, they brought in a psychiatrist and tried to schedule everybody for an half an hour visit. I don't remember it being a lifesaving experience. It might have been if, I had been more traumatized. They needed to do that, and maybe some people benefitted more than I. They could have said more to the group. There could have been more pulling us together as a group. There could have been a little more done. There could have been more gathering together as a family, letting feelings out, as a family and as a group. In the Philippines, they actually brought in a local organization, In Touch Foundation, a private volunteer organization staffed with psychiatrists and clinical social workers. They actually brought them in to deal with the post-traumatic feelings. That was more effective than a visit from one regional psychiatrist.

I don't remember talking to many people about it because they were on such a high. They were mostly colleagues, not family. Because we went right back to work immediately, I don't remember doing a whole lot of processing. I remember looking deeply into a lot of people's eyes and saying, are you o.k., and making sure in my own sense that they would be all right. I don't remember sitting down to counsel anybody or being counseled. So I think a number of people quite frankly may have suffered whatever reaction they may have had there because of going right back to work. They gave us an extraordinary two-week R&R a couple of weeks after the bombing. I thought it was a good thing. I needed to be with my family.

It was important for me to feel that I was o.k. So I didn't dwell on it and didn't want to dwell on it. I probably stuffed it some. But I knew my family was interested in hearing everything, every little detail, and I didn't feel it inappropriate to take up their time talking about it, whereas I would have felt that way with colleagues or acquaintances.

Malcolm arrived on Thursday after the bombing. I felt very shaken, but very strong at the same time. I had to hold it together and could because I wasn't physically hurt the way I had seen so many people, terribly physically hurt or dead. I felt like I was perfectly capable of doing what needed to be done and had a responsibility to do so. I didn't cry once until Malcolm arrived. I picked him up at the tarmac and he held me. That is when I cried for myself. The one other time I was upset was when I saw the Marine security guard. My experience would have been very different if I had been single. Malcolm was very important to me. I don't remember whether he asked a lot of questions or whether he just was there to listen when I needed help, but he was my sounding board. It gave me an appreciation of what we had to lose.

The bombing was less traumatic for me than the shelling of West Beirut later that August and early September. I had a much more sustained susceptibility to death. Shells were landing around us for thirty-six hours. I was feeling more mortal, because of what we had gone through four months before, and because there was more of a political breakdown. There was more threat out there. We were surrounded by Shiites and Phalangists and Druzes and everybody. There was more chaos outside.

I think that a little more could have been said about why they thought it had happened. Months afterwards we were still speculating who did it and why. They could have also addressed more forthrightly the degree of security that we did or did not have. There was a lot of resentment about the poor security. I also remember the administrative officer who was responsible for security moving on to some nice post. He was exonerated. Before the bombing, people had argued with him about needing to beef up the security. He had argued against it.

My sense is that our policy in the Middle East is horrendously imbalanced. Given I didn't know anything about the Middle East before serving in Lebanon, I may have developed this general disapproval about our policy from living there, but I really feel it viscerally now. Our policy is skewed, and our policy machinery is hostage to New York Congressmen and to specific Jewish-Americans and Jewish-American Israeli interests. I find myself fighting against being a bigot against Israel and the Congressmen.

My reaction has been for a long time that it was an almost inexpressible experience. I used to run into a lot of people who asked questions requiring either a ten-word answer or a two-hour answer. Most of the time I gave the ten-word answer. I felt like it required too much to go into to really convey the real feelings and the real experience. I wrote it all down. That was an important thing for me to get that down on ten legal-sized pages in a letter to my family.

For a couple of months, I saw the images of the morgue, the makeshift morgue, and would have to forcefully, willfully put them out of my mind. I never felt that they were any threat, not the way you feel scared about a scary movie, but it was just an unsettling image in my mind's eye. I don't really remember any others, probably because I was so intent on being all right afterwards.

I did deal with a little bit of survivor's guilt. I could not figure out, I was just absolutely consumed with trying to figure out, why I left the cafeteria early that day. Why was I healthy and others were dead? Why was Malcolm gone for the first time in six months? Why wasn't I deriving something more revelatory about myself? There should have been more beneficial knowledge coming out of that experience.

For most of my life I have tried to figure out what I believe about God and why we are here. I sort of honed my interest in figuring it out and in just absolutely revelling in being here. For six or seven years, I lived my life by trying to get the most out of it.

I think that it's not a bad idea to let people know in advance some basics about what they should expect in terms of their own personal reactions, their own human reactions to trauma. The overseas security course I went to focused on kidnapping and hostage situations, and nothing particularly relevant to that bombing experience.

Edited interview　　　　　Christine Crocker
January 5, 1994　　　　　Economic Officer Secretary in 1983

The bombing was near the end of our time in Beirut. There had been so many things prior to that in Lebanon, it was just one more horror.

I didn't hear the bomb. I did not hear it at all. I was in my office on the fourth floor, the Political Economic Section, sitting with my back to the windows, facing the center of the building, where the car came in. I saw the glow and felt the heat and the force of the wind. I thought we had been rocketed. I was thrown on top of my desk. I felt hot, real hot air and wind go across the back of my head. It was very quiet afterwards. You didn't hear people screaming. Everybody was so stunned. I heard Ryan saying, "Everybody get down, there could be a second one." Then I heard one of our TDYers who had been conked on the head by an air conditioner. That is when people started moving around. We first got this man down on the floor because he was really bleeding a lot. We got something to staunch the blood. The other secretary was also bleeding. She had been cut on her face. Dennis Foster was on the other side of the office. He had really gotten thrown. I just had some cuts and bruises.

We started down toward the other section. All I could see was daylight. That was really a strange, strange sensation. I walked down there with a feeling that I did not want to get there. I kept poking and looking into other places. I went into the hall looking into the main hallway of the building and trying to see where the other people were. Some were coming out of doors on the other side. People started filtering through and finding ways out through back windows, going down a couple of levels and then out of windows to the backyard. So we started moving people out from our office. Those not too badly hurt could function on their own. Dennis and I looked for a way out. It was hard to get across to the other side of the building. That section had gone down. There wasn't a lot of walking space. We got over to the other side just to see what the damage was like. A lot of people were filtering out from that side. I went back to my section. That's when we went to different floors to see how many people were dead. I got down to Personnel. That was the worst. They did not have Mylar[49] on their windows. Mary Apovian and Clemance Azouri had been sitting and having lunch in the front part of the office, which was right next to the center of the building. Their faces were ripped apart, but they could walk. Dennis and I got them out. We walked them across the rubble. We had to climb up and over on our side and managed to find a floor. The women could not see. Their faces were just hanging off. They could talk. They were so bewildered, it was fairly easy to move them around. By that time, people had set it up so they could help others through the window, down the ladder, across the yard, and up the ladder and out. There was a line of people.

Dennis and I went back into the building to continue searching. We collected the classified documents and secured the office. We knew the Lebanese Defense Forces were on the way and we had to get things locked up. I finally left the building about an hour later. Some people went down to shut down the boilers in the basement. I wasn't afraid.

It's funny. I really didn't think of it until later. It was shock, I'm sure. We were running on whatever. It took me a long time to actually think in terms of it, because after leaving the Embassy I went with Diane Dillard and Lisa Piascik on a body search. We went first to the French hospital, but they didn't have any Americans. They did clean up my little wounds. From there we went to AUH.

The first thing they asked us to do was go to the morgue. It really wasn't that bad. It's worse thinking about it now. We just identified people. Some of them we didn't know. There was a guy in a uniform who had his ID, and Bill McIntyre was there, too. Some looked normal. Some were bloated and decomposed. It's very strange. Of course, the morgue wasn't prepared. Obviously, they had other corpses. They had some that were already put in lockers, and others were just on a table and stretchers. It was too crowded. They were allowing too many people in and out. They got it cleared up and did a good job.

Then we went to the hospital. It was so tough because there were people in the halls. They seemed to be moving people as quickly as they could.

In some ways, Sabra-Shatila was almost worst [sic]. Having been in Beirut for a while, I had seen an occasional dead body, but this was just one of the most unbelievable things. The bombing was terrible, just dreadful, but Sabra-Shatila stands out for me. It was the first time I ever realized people could be that way. Doing those things. Of course, I understand intellectually, but it was pretty horrible. At the time when you first encounter it, it's not as horrifying as it should be. It isn't. You don't gag. You don't start crying or wringing your hands or anything. It's later, of course, when it really gets you.

I left AUH and finally went home. I still had glass in my hair. I was kind of bloody. It was then I remember being absolutely terrified to be home by myself. It took me the longest time to get over. I don't think it left me for a long time, even when we were back in the States. A lot of people said that being home alone was hard. Not so much frightening. A few of the single women said it really didn't bother them. They didn't feel any different than they did before about being home by themselves. I've never seen dead people before and I couldn't stand the aloneness.

Throughout that night we couldn't sleep. We actually did try. We got in bed and tried to get some sleep. But we could not and got back up and went back down to the Embassy. They were still getting people out and we were there all night. Then the Marines raised the flag. Probably that was when I first cried.

I can't remember when it dawned on me that all of these people had been killed, when I first felt it. It may have been far later than that. I also had a fear of windows. There were just some things that didn't all end in Beirut.

One of the things that happened not too long after—in June—was the earthquake. It was early morning and [it] woke us up. Both Ryan and I thought, "We've been hit." Another time, when there was fighting around the British Embassy and a shell hit nearby, somebody in the office said I threw myself forward on the desk and said, "Whew." I remember feeling hot air on the back of my neck. I was thinking, "I didn't hear the car bomb, but I heard the shell." I remember thinking, well, that's just weird, because I know consciously I did not hear it.

I'm sure the bombing must have been in some way very important in what went on later, but I can't pinpoint it. When we went back to Beirut when Ryan was Ambassador, nothing surprised me. What people did to each other. The way they talked about each other no longer shocked me. Maybe it hardened me more than changed my philosophy. Maybe I have a lot less faith in mankind now. You know that you could not do these things, and yet obviously people can do them. I don't know about myself maybe as clearly as I think I do. Who knows any more? Maybe I'm even more unwilling to ever allow anything like that to happen. I don't know. I've never been put to the test.

In some ways I'm probably more foolhardy. I was never frightened in Beirut this time. I never really worried about it. I worried about Ryan, but I really never worried about me. I've never been a strong believer in fate but...I can't stand the idea that some force back there has all that control and that I don't.

I was going to talk to the psychiatrist, but it was just one of those things. I just ended up not having time. People got their lives back to normal as quickly as they could and did what they could. We had to set up more offices, get the Marines a new place to live, and all those things. People got back to work. It was good. Important that they did it.

People did feel a little bit more tense about their lives. One of the nights when the Marines were still living in the basement parking lot, they had us to dinner. No one talked about the bombing until late in the evening when they had had too much to drink. Then there was some tussling, a little bit of talk about the bombing, but then people were angry. That was interesting. People got angry with each other for a while. It blew up. It blew over. They never said anything specific. I think it was a reaction. People, mostly the Marines, were just angry.

The Embassy handled the memorial service at the AUB chapel well. I must say Bob Pugh was really helpful. Bob Dillon spoke. So did a Shiia, a Sunni and a Christian. Bob Dillon lost it toward the end, and that just broke everybody up. It was a good thing.

We didn't go on our R&R right away. We kept trying to get out of it. We did not want to go to Washington, because it would not have been useful. But they were giving tickets to Washington. We went for a day and went to Ireland. It was the right place for us to go.

Eagleburger came out and he accompanied the bodies back. They sent out their little cast of characters. All it did was create more work. But it was the right thing and Washington had to do it.

Security sent out questionnaires asking us about what we heard, saw, felt. It was directed at the bombing itself. They of course had people who came out early on to see what the bomb was and how big it was. They talked to people.

We had one couple who did leave post. Washington sent its delegation out. Everyone could choose to leave immediately. Nothing would go in their record. They would just try and find them good assignments.

The bombing changed the way we functioned. That really altered every embassy in the world. Whether we like it or not, so many of us work in a fortress. Our security has become top, top, top, priority. Whether that's good or not, I don't know. Foreign Service Officers will never have the type of experiences we had early on in our careers when going across the desert wildly, mindlessly, and other adventures were possible.

FSI asked me to talk to the Foreign Service secretaries. Ordinarily FSI gives us some things to specifically mention. I have done it with incoming secretaries. I've gone to speak to them. You don't really give speeches for the most part. It's focused mostly on questions. They've always wanted to hear about Beirut. I've never gone into great detail about bombings, and massacres, and things, but let them know that there is danger out there.

I think the two-day briefing is a good course and I really do think that people in this day have to keep aware. I don't know anything about the training videos.

The bombing is one of those events that you think about on a fairly regular basis. For an unknown reason, I don't know why, it's something I think about a lot. I don't know how to change that. Deep down change that. I can't tell you exactly why. I don't think it's made me a better person. I know that if it ever happened to me again I could still carry on. It makes you feel pretty good about yourself. I don't completely fall to pieces. That is rather reassuring. It's funny because I would think, how could I have known that if I hadn't been there?

The Embassy was bombed because we couldn't believe that it would happen. Who in their right mind would have been in a truck and driven into the Marine barracks with all these fences? All these guns. Nobody used them and yet, you know, there he goes right in there. Who would have thought? I still think, who could hate that much?

Edited interview Ryan Crocker
January 4, 1994 Political Officer in 1983

I was in my office, which was on the northeastern corner of [the] fourth floor of the wing that was bombed, but on the back side of the building. I was at my desk when it went off. I saw a flash of light from the balcony in the outer office. My initial assumption was that our suite of offices had been hit by a RPG or a rocket. The force of the explosion carried through our offices. Within fifty seconds or so, I went into the outer office to check on people. I could see through the outer doors of the suite that the offices on the corniche side of the corridor were simply no longer there. I was staring out into space. I realized immediately that we had been the target of a major bomb.

Certain chemical reactions took over. I was, and all those around me were, extremely calm, including those injured. Time seemed to move in very, very slow motion. A very methodical process of looking after the injured and moving people out got underway. When that was in hand, the next thing I did was to determine whether or not we still had an ambassador and DCM, or, God forbid, that I might be in charge. I went off to look into that and encountered both of them coming down the central staircase. After I saw Bob Pugh and Bob Dillon, I joined with one of the Marines and checked through the various floors. We went down to see if anything could be done for the Marines in Post One. Various chemical reactions tended to keep us calm, carrying us straight through dovetailing with exhaustion. We went several nights without sleep, supervising the search and recovery of bodies. I don't recall any particular emotional spikes. People just sort of did what came naturally. Diane, of course, took over trying to account for people. A lot of people were checking on information which was circulating around. For a while, I kept a list, based on the Embassy phone listing, of people who had been seen and people who had not been seen. That kind of thing. That probably went on for three or four hours.

I encountered Jack Massengill, the Marine, and we did a sweep of the Embassy. We went to the upper floors and then went down into the main lobby area, looking for Post One. The enormity of what had happened was clear, because *that* was like walking into hell. It was pitch black. The face of the building had collapsed in on the lobby and fires were burning inside. It was very clear that no one in that area could possibly have survived. By the time I got to the Consular Section, the Marines, rescue workers, and the French were there. The initial emergency recovery was in hand.

What I did was probably the best possible way of dealing with the emotional and psychological impact of that kind of thing. I just physically wore myself out, and when I did get a good night's sleep, I was right back at it. I felt tremendous demands placed on me and was doing a lot of the night shift work on the recovery operation. We still had the negotiation in process. Remember, it was several weeks later that the May 17 agreement was signed and Morrie Draper needed things. We had to analyze the impact of the bombing on our situation in Lebanon and on the Lebanese political fabric. It was a blur of intense activity. Sleeplessness was just your life. I couldn't just crawl into bed. That was probably very good medicine. I think it is very important when you come out of something like that to have a sense that what you did was important and that you are not some shattered survivor, wandering aimlessly in a field of battle. You had a mission.

There was a woman psychiatrist, I think she was military.

We were all encouraged, indeed directed, to see her. She was very pleasant, very level-headed. She was good in the sense that she was not demanding that you unveil a crisis to her. If you were feeling o.k., it was fine with her. I had a very brief conversation with her. Generally speaking, I thought it was nice that they sent in a psychiatrist. I didn't really feel the need then or afterwards to talk to one.

We had an R&R, and it was a bizarre episode. You had to be gone for at least a week, so we came all the way back to Washington and showed up in the NEA. It was a device to get people out.

I pretty much put the bombing in the larger frame of events in Lebanon. In the aftermath of the 1982 Israeli invasion, we had become not simply observers, chroniclers of the debacle, but very much leading participants. That took us from the profile and risk level we had since

1975 and gave us an entirely new risk factor, commensurate with our much larger role. We became one with others who suffered similarly: Iraqis, Palestinians, the Syrians, and on occasion Lebanese factions. The obvious connection between our bombing and the bombing six months later of the Marine barracks, I think, bears that out. I see the bombing as a political act of terror and one very much of the general fabric of the times. Again, as bad as it was, it wasn't the only event: the Israeli invasion itself, the Sabra-Shatila massacres, and the attempted takeover of West Beirut by the militia in 1983 which we were caught up in. Our military training team was in [sic] particularly grave risk for a 48-hour period. The bombing became a part of rather a long three-year time of trial.

I don't think anyone can live through something like the bombing without having it affect them. It certainly made me very glad to be alive. I occasionally use that as a reference point when other much smaller events are preoccupying me or concerning me. It helps to look back and remember what you've been through. To go through it, you simply are different on the other end. I am a more mature person than I might otherwise be. I think I have a sense of what the world can do to you if you are not careful. And I have something else that is valuable. I know that I can deal with horror. I've been through it. Again I have the sense, it is very, very nice to still smell the daisies.

Going back to Beirut as Ambassador, one rather obvious goal I set for myself was that we would not be the object of a car bomb or any other major attack. We would have every means whatsoever of preventing it and be extremely methodical in going over our security. We went over and over it and over again. It was a real issue and not a theoretical one. We did innumerable "what if's," and set up "bad teams." You are the enemy and you are going to blow us up. How are you going to do it? I asked the staff to construct a means of attack in the compound. I involved the entire staff, not just the security staff. It's a game anybody can and should play. You are equally likely to die by a car bomb if you are a political officer or a security officer. It behooves us all to think through possible vulnerabilities. We often discussed security-related issues at general staff meetings simply because they did apply to everybody.

The other thing that I think is so important, and not just for the crisis of the moment, but in a long drawn-out crisis environment, is the ability to be calm. Maintain perspective, keep your attention focused out, not just on yourself. And keep a sense of humor.

There are two things I think we need to do. First is make people aware of the fact that new world order is very much new world disorder in terms of threat, and that they have to think about it and take responsibility for thinking about it. They can't simply look to other forces or elements to protect them from danger. But the second thing is to mitigate that by making it simply part of our life, not to scare people with it, but to go over it so often that it becomes normal, so that people are not frightened by the idea of thinking about risk and threat and danger. Part of our overseas role should be to demystify danger.

When we got back to Beirut, we organized a service for the anniversary in April 1991. We built a memorial garden with a plaque of names of all of those who were killed. It was all done by volunteers. Each April 18 from 1991 to 1993, we had a memorial ceremony. Last year for the tenth anniversary we made it rather a bigger deal. The Commandant of the Marine Corps sent out an honor guard. We told the Department that this was the tenth anniversary of the most catastrophic event in American diplomatic custodian history, and we were going to commemorate it out there. We invited all of the Foreign Service national retirees and the families of the Lebanese who were killed in the bombing. I had suggested that an appropriate statement in the name of the Secretary of State be read. In fact, I encountered bureaucratic resistance back in Washington. "Let's just bury the past." But I finally did get a statement after they learned that Commandant of the Marine Corps had sent a statement. The Lebanese appreciated the commemoration, which was extremely difficult to get through if you had a speaking role. They seemed to find it very therapeutic. There was a tremendous amount of crying and general sorrow. I think it helped them to come to terms with the bombing and to realize that we do care and remember what happened out there.

There was a practical consequence, too. We took the occasion to get the Workmen's Compensation cases straightened out. It was awful. Many survivors who had run into bureaucratic tangles were not getting compensation checks. They couldn't move the system. We simply took the occasion to say, we are going to do this. I was not going to stand there in front of these people and say how much we care about the sacrifices their loved ones had made and not even settle those back cases.

Every year, starting from the first year, Christine and I always send an anonymous basket of carnations to the 23rd Street entrance of the State Department. We have a standing order with the florist. The flowers are placed under the plaque of those who were killed in service.

Why weren't we more prepared for the bombing than we were? It hadn't happened before. It is very difficult to understand what may happen to you if you don't have some kind of experiential base to deal with, and massive suicide bomb attacks on American Embassies just simply were not part of the inventory. Many of us felt nervous out there. Because of 1982, we were at greater risk than before, but I doubt if anyone foresaw that kind of massive bomb attack. We were worried about assassinations, rocket attacks, the usual inventory in Lebanon, but not that. The irony was, there had been a precedent: the December 1981 bombing of the Iraqi Embassy. It was completely leveled. A car had gotten into its underground parking garage, as far as we could tell. But that was the Iraqis. They were an endangered species in Lebanon anyway, with a history of that kind of thing. I don't think we ever put the one together with the other in relation to ourselves.

At the end of last year, I was over at FSI with the new A 100 class. The course director asked me to talk about these things: coping with crisis, how to deal with the inevitable threats, risks, dangers, and crises that the Foreign Service will give out to you in the course of a career. I was asked to make it purely practical, drawing from experience. I told them that virtually every single officer in the room, if she or he pursues a fifteen- or twenty-year stint in the State Department (assuming that they don't spend it all in Western Europe) would see almost without doubt shots fired in anger, witness an evacuation in some form or other—dependents or personnel—and would be in a crisis of some magnitude. That is simply the way of the world. To go through the ways in which you can prepare yourself can help wonderfully. When you know you are going into a tense area, imagine the various scenarios that could be functional and ask yourself how you would deal with them or how the mission would deal with them. If you are pre-programmed in some way, it can help immeasurably in getting your bearings in the first minutes of an unexpected disaster. They have "Coping with Violence Abroad," which is fast-paced. It probably sensitizes you to the fact that the world is a dangerous place. I don't think it takes you to the next step, which is to normalize the danger, which isn't to scare you from going overseas. Be aware of danger to be able to deal with it, not to be terrified of it.

Edited interview   Diane Dillard
February 14, 1994   Consular Section Chief in 1983

I'd gotten a call from the DCM about five of one saying that somebody from the palace was going to come and see me at one-thirty, so I hurried home for lunch and to walk my dog. I was heating some soup and suddenly a tremendous crack of thunder, I thought, sounded. It really hurt my ears. After a minute the windows fell in. Then I realized it wasn't thunder. I went to the phone to call my family, because I knew whatever it was, I didn't know what it was, they would hear about it and I'd better tell them that I was all right. The line was dead. I went across to my neighbor's apartment thinking she might know what was happening. Just then the DCM's wife came downstairs and said it was the Embassy. We looked out my neighbor's window, which faced in the direction of the Embassy. You could see smoke coming up, but the building itself looked fine. I had no idea what the front of the building looked like from there. I went on down to the Embassy. People started coming out of the back of the Embassy. There were some wounded that I helped find a place to sit down. When I went around to the front of the building for the first time, I could see a great hunk of my section was gone. Two-thirds of my office was gone. I thought, well, I'll have to think about that later. Then I realized that the cafeteria was gone and that you and Bob were in there. I thought, well, you're dead, but I'll just have to think about that after a while. Then the DCM directed me to track down everybody. Shortly after that we heard that the wounded were being taken to the French compound in East Beirut. One of the Marine doctors got a jeep for us: Lisa Piascik, Christine Crocker, and me. We went against a horrendous flow of traffic. We could hardly get by because everybody was coming down to see [the Embassy]. We got to the hospital and waited, but nobody came. The doctor treated Christine's cuts. It was a rest spot for us to gather ourselves. We went back to the American University Hospital to find out who was there. They did give me a preliminary list and I saw that you were there. I was very surprised and, needless to say, pleased. The doctors came in and asked me to go to the morgue and to identify an employee, the husband of a Lebanese woman. It was very hard at first to figure out anybody, because they were covered with a gray dust. I guess when a building goes there is a lot of cement dust. When people are lying down, for some reason, it's harder to tell who they are. I looked around through the bodies and saw one which I believed was her husband because he had kind of squared off teeth. The top of his head was blown off and his insides were hanging out, so I asked them to put something over his head and over his middle before they showed her the body. She said no, that wasn't her husband. I thought well, if that's not her husband, I really can't do this job. It turned out that it was her husband. They found something in his pocket. I spent a lot of time in the morgue trying to identify the people. Some of them I hadn't known. Some were there on TDY. They had a name on one person which I knew was not right. I went into another room and I found the person with that name. This went on for all that week. The Department wanted to bring a planeload of people out. Under Secretary [for Political Affairs, Department of State] Eagleburger wanted to come on a Wednesday and leave on Thursday. I knew that wasn't going to work but couldn't figure out why. Finally it dawned on me that we would not have all the bodies yet. So they agreed to come on Friday and leave on Saturday. On Friday at five-thirty, we found the last body.

The Saturday after the bombing we had a ceremony to see the bodies off onto the plane. Then we came back and started working. The crisis wasn't over. It was just more intense. The big shots had come and gone. We still had to do the work and that was really hard.

I was withdrawn in a way. I was more an observer than a participant in life at that point. I walked my dog along the corniche every afternoon for about forty-five minutes. It was so intense, I needed to be alone to try to come to grips with things. We didn't have any time to sleep or anything. I tried to make myself cry. I felt I should cry. It was very good for me to do that. I don't know how I knew to do that but it helped me a lot. We got very little sleep. I remember on Tuesday the Public Affairs Officer came to my house. He was very concerned about the people in the library who worked for him. He was agitated and he had been hurt. I said, "You must be exhausted." He said, "Yeah, I only got five hours sleep." I thought, five hours sleep, how wonderful!

I was exhausted. My adrenaline kept me going all the time I was assigned there, but the minute I left Lebanon, I fell apart. Just about the time I was recovering, they blew up the Annex. That was even harder. I did not really recover from the whole experience of Beirut while I was there. I had this feeling, particularly when we were living in the compound, that when I was away something was going to happen to the people there. I always felt very uneasy being away from the compound. It was stupid. Intellectually, it was crazy, but I couldn't help it. I had to hurry back there so they'd be all right.

The regional medical doctor came out. I think we had two doctors. A psychiatrist came on the plane from Washington. I assume he talked to everybody. He talked to me. I know that he talked to some others. I enjoyed talking to him. It was helpful to me. He had a very commonsense approach. A couple of weeks after that, they sent another psychiatrist in to talk to groups and individuals.

When I went on R&R, I was really exhausted. I slept a lot. It was very good for me. Unfortunately, I waited too long to go on the next R&R, so I was all beat up again. My adrenaline kept me going, but once I finished altogether with Beirut, I was completely wiped out.

The bombing is part of my history. I find myself talking about things in Beirut. I probably shouldn't, because people aren't really that interested. It's not that it was wonderful to be there in the bombing, it's just that it's part of my life and it's interesting, I think, but I have to be careful. I've talked to a few colleagues who were there. I think we are all kind of tired of it. There is danger wherever you go now. For many people in the Foreign Service, danger has become more commonplace. You just feel like people don't really want to talk about these things. I've talked with people that lived through it, because we were all there, living together. The bombing was the worst thing that happened to the Embassy family, but it wasn't the end of crisis. Every day was kind of a crisis. We were shelled a lot. The bombing was like the beginning. I had thought until about mid-July that things were going to be better. Then it started disintegrating. We had the war of August 29, 30, 31 and then we had the war of October 7 and 8. Dependents would be sent off to Cyprus, and then we ended up living in a compound because people were being kidnapped. Then the Marine bombing happened. That's when I finally broke down. I couldn't stop crying. The French military had been bombed at the same time. I finally pulled myself together and went over there to see if I could help.

I was very fortunate. I thought I was in Beirut for a purpose, that it was all God's plan that I be there. Having to walk my dog meant I was out of the building when it happened, so I didn't suffer the shock of the explosion. That put me way ahead of everybody else, because they all had undergone this physical experience. I always believed that God was using me. It gave me a reason for being there. I don't know why the bombing happened. I just had a sense that I was there as a part of God's plan. I was there to do that job and being out of the Embassy prepared me to do the job.

When I went to Florence in the fall of 1985, I was very concerned about the building, because our building in Beirut had been so vulnerable. In Italy we were right on the street. I finally got the Embassy in Rome and the City Government to let us put up a barrier. Once that happened, I forgot about it. I had done all I could do to protect the building and employees. But until then I was always sure I was going to come around the corner and see it blow up.

When I was on R&R in London, everyone was wonderful. I probably looked a little wretched. A friend, a local hire who worked in the consular section, Shirley, sat me down and said, "Tell me all about it." When I told her that people looked like statues, all covered in gray dust, she said, "Yes, that's what it's like." When I told her some of the decisions that I made in Beirut, she said, "Yes, that is what I would have done." She gave me a reference point. She was older and had experience during World War II. It was wonderful talking to someone who knew about death and dying. Shirley sought me out to talk to me. It made me feel better knowing how others reacted. That's why I did the tape. I wanted to help others, to let them know how people think. It would have been nice to talk with someone in the Department, but I didn't know anyone. No one sought me out.

I think the Embassy was bombed because they were trying to kill the Ambassador, who was the symbol of America. They wanted to show that they were better than we were. I gathered that the Syrians were behind the bombing. There was a Palestinian who worked as a porter at the Embassy who was involved in it, so it wasn't strictly a nationalist thing. It was a group that didn't like us. One could think that it might have been the Israelis, because the Israelis seemed not to have wanted stability in that part of the world at that point.

I wasn't prepared at all. It was the first time we had ever had that kind of operation. We have a much better program now. A lot has been learned. It wasn't learned right away, but I think the tapes that they did on crisis and how to help other people in a crisis situation have been most useful. I think they have a good program. For example, they have a good evacuation program. They have a fly-away team that can go out with satellite phones and things like that to assist embassies in crisis. I think that was one of the things that came out of the Beirut bombing. We did get help, but it was kind of *ad hoc*. It wasn't very organized, and you had to kind of fight to get the help you needed. We could have used the eye of someone coming in from outside. Older, more experienced officers should be on the fly- away team.

Making the video "Crisis Work, Crisis Worker" was very good for me. Before I went to Florence, I talked to Sheila Platt. When I came back for the filming, I also spent a lot of time with Marilyn Holmes discussing things. I was a little worried about it before I started the filming. I hadn't really talked about those things with anybody. In the filming Sheila would bring up things that I had said to her the summer before and that I had forgotten. I realized that, actually, I was getting over it and putting it behind me. It was very positive for me to get to do that video. I shared my feelings because I thought that would be helpful to other people. It wasn't until I saw the tape in the fall of 1985 that I understood that what I had experienced was a kind of shock. They called it denial, a stress reaction. Denial is an all right kind of stress reaction to have. I was glad to know that was not unique to me.

Edited interview Robert Dillon
January 19, 1994 Ambassador in 1983

I was in my office when the bomb went off at five after one. I was getting ready to go out and jog. I had just been talking with one of the bodyguards, a chauffeur, and my Lebanese social secretary. It was horrible. She was killed. I had a phone call that morning from a German banker, a nice guy. At the very last minute I decided I would return the call. I was standing in front of the window, eight floors up, phone in hand. I had one of those heavy Marine T-shirts that someone had given me, and I was trying to put it on at the same time I made the call. In the meantime, the others had already gone down. It was great luck that my arms were in front of my face and I had that heavy T-shirt. The window blew in. I fell on my back. I never heard a sound. I never heard anything. Other people said it was the loudest explosion they had ever heard, but anyhow I never heard it. Perhaps I was unconscious for a short time. I don't think so. I was on my back bewildered, angry, cursing. The brick wall behind my desk blew out very slowly and collapsed across me and a large flag. There was a chair and a flagstaff which eased the fall. From the waist down, I was covered with rubble. I thought we had been hit by a rocket, because a week or so before, another part of the building had been hit by an RPG, a rocket-propelled grenade. I mention this simply because it's interesting about people. We are so self-centered. When this happened, I'm not lying there thinking of the terrible tragedy that has occurred: lots of people have been killed, the United States has been damaged. I'm lying there thinking, "My God, those so-and-sos almost got me that time," because I thought a rocket had hit my office. Bob Pugh and Dorothy Pascoe came in looking a little disheveled. They grabbed the flagstaff and pried the brick wall off my body and I got out. I thought my legs had been crushed, because I was numb. I was relieved to find out that they weren't. I suffered literally no injuries. My arms were filled with glass. For several days thereafter, the stuff would keep coming out. My legs were bruised and a few cuts, but no serious injury. The office then filled up with smoke and tear gas, because the tear gas grenades in the lobby were set off. Bob Pugh started terrible coughing, and we got to a window with a ledge, not a thin ledge, something we could stand on, and we got out the window actually where we could breathe. A breeze came up and blew everything away. The central stairway and the elevator, obviously, were gone but there was a stairway on another wing and we made our way over there. Rubble was everywhere. We started down and only then understood what had happened. I remarked fatuously to somebody as we were going down a floor, "My God, I bet somebody was hurt down here." We went down a few more floors and the destruction was greater. At first it didn't occur to us that people had been killed. We realized there had been some serious injuries. We got down to the third or second floor and somebody ran up to me to say Bill McIntyre was dead. Then I noticed Mary Lee McIntyre sitting there with blood streaming down her face. I picked her up and took her to a window and handed her to somebody.

Typical of the Foreign Service, we began to report. We put together very quickly a list of the people we believed had been in the building. Instead of trying to report to Washington who was dead, we were reporting who was alive. For an hour or so it was quite positive, because we were checking off a lot of names. After about an hour, we stopped and looked at the gaps in the list. You think, my God, this has really been awful. The last person brought out alive as far as I know was Mr. Copti. It was about five hours afterwards.

A few bodies were brought out, and then, of course, you just find scraps and pieces. You identify people through toes or boots. When they brought you out, Anne, I happened to be standing there. You looked like a piece of hamburger, you really did. You looked terrible. The two people I remember were you and Copti.

My mother and my wife were just a few blocks away from the Embassy. Thank God they hadn't come into the Embassy. They were playing bridge. I think if they had not been in Beirut they would have been terrified. But they were there and we lived through it together.

We got so busy, I supposed that was what saved us. I think combat is like that. You're so busy doing what you're doing that you don't have time to reflect on the horror. I think that's what happened to all of us. It was several days before I started thinking about what a horrible thing had happened. I didn't cry until I talked in the chapel at AUB probably a week or ten days later. The families, most of them

Lebanese, of course, and a few American families were there for people who had lost their relatives. John Reid, who was a great help throughout this thing, had helped me put together a little talk. I stood up there and looked down at all these people who were hanging on every word. Of course, they wanted to hear that their loved ones had died for some reason. I'm standing there thinking, those people didn't die for any reason. There's a flawed U.S. policy. You know all the history, our involvement in the Middle East, everything that has happened. What I was feeling was the insanity of the actual perpetrators, to feel that by murdering sixty-three people they would make the world a better place. I was down to about the last sentence or two and I just couldn't go on. I don't think I sobbed, but tears welled up. I just stopped. That was the first time I really felt emotionally overwhelmed by the bombing. It was a very emotional moment.

The personnel people at the Department of State reacted very quickly. Everybody wanted to be helpful. They sent somebody up to help us in dealing with the local employees. The number two in CIA came out immediately. The military is good in this kind of thing. They've been doing it for two centuries. They understand how to deal with death, injury, bereaved families.

So much happened after that. The bombing was a very dramatic incident, and on one level I'm still angry. But, I can't say that I was emotionally any more bothered by that than I was over Sabra-Shatila. I left a few days before the Marine bombing, but those pictures bothered me a great deal. I've been through a couple of other things. One of them was a giant bomb. It was like a huge door slamming behind me. I dreamed of that one. I don't know if explosions frighten me now, but I feel apprehensive when I hear an explosion.

I had a kind of recurrent reaction, one of sadness. I would think of this thing and feel immensely, immensely sad. And then anger. Sadness, anger, sadness, anger. I don't know whether that is a normal reaction or not. They rushed a psychologist out, he could have been a psychiatrist, from the State Department to talk to all the survivors. I had talked to him once before during a terrorist incident in Malaysia in 1975, when the Japanese Red Army took over part of the Embassy. The psychologist asked me how I felt. I said, I don't understand it. I feel normal. We have all been so busy all the time that I really didn't think about what happened. I think about what we're doing and when it's time to go to sleep, I go to sleep. I wondered if something were wrong. Is this a natural human reaction? The guy told me these were normal reactions, because psychologically we put up defenses or we couldn't live through these things. They would destroy us. It had, I think, an impact on my view of my life. Occasionally, when Sue and I are discouraged about something we look at each other and say, well, what the hell, we're alive. It has enabled me to be more philosophical than I ever was. It makes you perhaps more compassionate. I think I was a compassionate person already, but it takes you in that direction. It is not the bombing alone that made me decide—I was very slow in deciding—I wanted to leave the Foreign Service, but the whole Beirut experience. In fact it was a very sour experience, and that was the reason I went to the U.N.

Later, the blowing up of the Embassy got all mixed up with other things that I'm angry about. See, I'm still angry about the bombing. I'm angry about the stupidity of it all. I'm angry about all the ambitious bastards who flooded into Beirut while we were trying to cope with things. I'm angry about our absolute cowardice in not facing up to the Israelis and what they were doing. I'm angry about Sabra-Shatila. I'm angry about Ain Helway.[50] You and I went through Ain Helway after it had been flattened. I saw Ain Helway several times. I saw it just before the Israeli invasion. I saw it just afterwards, and I saw it when the rubble had simply been bulldozed away. I remember picking up a newspaper and reading that a group of retired American military officers had been brought up by bus from Israel, escorted by the Israelis, and looked at everything. They didn't see any damage, which just outraged me. Didn't see any damage! They went right through Ain Helway, which was a town with 50,000 people. It was just a flat field now. These guys didn't see anything because they didn't know what had been there before. That really outraged me. Sabra-Shatila and parts of Ain Helway stunk with rotting bodies that had just been bulldozed over. As I remember all of this stuff, I remember being up in Baabda when some Israeli tourists arrived. They were in shorts and very trim and stylish in sport shirts. Half a million people three miles away were suffering.

Then there was my whole relationship with the NSC staff. I'd gotten on quite well with Phil Habib, Morris Draper, and Chris Ross, the special envoy group. We sometimes had shouting arguments, but we never lied to each other. Then the NSC staff crowd headed by Bud McFarland came in. These people were secretive and wrong on all sorts of things. When I think about all of that, I wonder if Foreign Service Officers ever focus on the human side of things. I never went back to the Foreign Service.

We were targeted by the Shiite group, Hizballah. It was the Musawi family over in the Bekaa that apparently did it. I've seen an interview on BBC with Musawi quite recently. He denied that they had done it and then told why they had done it. The Shiites were outraged by the Israeli invasion of Lebanon. They were outraged that they were in the hands of the Israelis and had long held grievances against the Maronite Christians in Lebanon. They saw us as the pillar of support, going along with all of these people. They believed that perhaps we had put the Israelis up to the invasion which, of course, we didn't. On the other hand, we did foolish things. After the invasion, Congress voted to increase military aid to the Israelis. People aren't stupid; yes, they do look at the world differently, but they're not stupid. They decided that we were their enemies. The idea of a blow against the greatest nation in the world was something that appealed to them very strongly and something that people were willing to give their lives for and they did. It was a suicide attack. From their point of view, we had become the enemy. We didn't see it that way. We never do. We didn't see it that way. We didn't think of those people as our enemies. I think the people who planned and carried out the attack did it as a political gesture. The idea that the downtrodden could inflict major injury on the greatest power on earth was very important. Well, it's interesting, you see, you're sitting there in the American Embassy in Lebanon. You're angry about the invasion. You've opposed it. You've made it clear to your government, one hopes at all levels, that the Israelis had lied about their plans. They've lied about their execution. They've lied about everything. The Israelis, of course, pegged us, and me in particular, as somehow being pretty unfriendly to them. It doesn't give you any immunity, but it makes it harder for you to believe that the Lebanese are going to want to kill sixty-three of you. The other thing that had happened on the ground was that physically we had lost our defenses. We hadn't realized it. We used to be right on the cusp between a Druze-held area and a PLO-held area. The PLO and the Druze militia protected us not for humanitarian reasons, but for political reasons. They had a stake in our presence. I think we were slow to understand the consequences of having been shorn of all that protection and that we were on our own resources. We were very vulnerable. We understood that. There had been car bombs all over the place. We reacted to that. We had cleared out the area around the Embassy. A car couldn't stop, for instance, and an abandoned car was destroyed. The possibility of a suicide attack was understood, and we had ordered some barriers to be put up. Some ram-proof barriers had just arrived but weren't up. There is another level, it makes you sound like a boob, but there is another level at which you don't realize how vulnerable you really are. Americans can and do engage in suicidal attacks [in terms of disregarding danger]. This is part of our culture. You realize that your chances of being killed are very high on a suicidal attack. We don't engage in suicide attacks [i.e., t]he kamikaze idea is just so foreign to our culture that we talk about it in the abstract. It's no longer abstract, but in 1983 a suicide attack was a very abstract idea still. We had one example, and we weren't even sure of that. The Iraqi Embassy was destroyed. Nobody knew what had happened, but we speculated that it had been a suicide attack. The first time we really knew that these people, in fact, would engage in suicide attacks was when our Embassy was destroyed. I understand that the Musawi backed by the Iranians were involved. I don't know that anybody had any information to directly implicate the Syrians; on the other hand, neither the Musawis nor the Iranians could have operated without at least Syrian acquiescence, because both operated right out of Syrian-controlled Bekaa.

I'm troubled, indeed saddened, by the defenses behind which our people live. Embassies look like giant prisons. They're big fortresses. Isolated. And yet I remind myself that if we had had something like that in Lebanon, we would have been secure. Secure and they could not have blown up the Embassy. If anyone wants to pursue a Foreign Service life, this is part of it. It's like being in the Army. There isn't any safe way to do it. If the danger of terrorism makes it impossible for you to go out and interact with other people, you'd better not do it.

This is perhaps a minor point, but one that occurred to me. I certainly believed in spouses going. It's very important that spouses share danger. It was important personally that Sue and I have shared a lot of the danger in Lebanon. It made it far easier for me to adjust after that than after some experiences during the Korean War, which I didn't share with anybody. I always had the feeling my family never understood. On a political level, I do not and have never felt that we should retreat from the Middle East. I believe that we have to behave like sensible adults, which is very difficult for Americans, and do our best to solve at least the most important problem, which is the Palestinian problem, and that we not let ourselves be bullied by the Israelis and their friends into doing things against our interest. I certainly do not think that we can flip over and toady to Arab tyrants and become outrageously anti-Israel. But we behaved so foolishly and there's been such a thing of silence.

Edited interview　　　　　　Dick Gannon
January 11, 1994　　　　　　Security Officer in 1983

I have very mixed emotions about my assignment to Beirut, and certainly the bombing was the low point, as far as I was concerned, with regard to the ten months that I spent in the country. I think the U.S. government went into Beirut with the best of intentions in terms of trying to help the Lebanese establish a legitimate government. We had military forces there to try and buy time for the Lebanese to rebuild their military, so that they could control the situation in the country, but overall I would have to say that I think, and this is with benefit of hindsight, that U.S. intervention there was very naive. We did not have, in my view, a full appreciation for the nuances of the situation, for the cultural differences, and our lack of a cohesive policy, with regard to not just Lebanon but the Middle East, has repeatedly gotten us into trouble. I don't think the U.S. policy with regard to Lebanon was well-founded. I think it was basically a policy which was not thought out and which resulted in a terrible, terrible series of tragedies: bombing of the Embassy, the bombing of the Marine barracks and then a second bombing of the Embassy. So I think the

U.S. went in with good intentions, but not fully realizing the complexity of the situation and not having a full understanding of what the ramifications of U.S. involvement might be.

My experience there was not my view of a positive experience at all, but you have to understand that I've had additional experience in the way the Middle East has touched me. Quite honestly, I would not be inclined to serve in the Middle East again. It would have to be a very compelling argument for me to change my position. My younger brother was on the Pan Am flight coming out of Beirut. Beirut, Lebanon, has touched me very personally.

It isn't something that I have been able to resolve easily and not something that I would engage in again.

I was in my office on the first floor and talking to a colleague, Dave Roberts, who had flown in from Casablanca. He wanted to talk to me about certain aspects of the program. My comment to Dave was, "Have you had lunch yet?" He said, "Yes," and I said, "Well, we might as well start out in here," and we sat down in the security office on the first floor right at 1:00. It was only a few minutes later when the blast occurred. At the time, I was seated behind a large standard government desk. The blast actually shook the building. I suppose we were knocked over, because we both ended up on the floor. I recall saying, "Stay down, stay down," fearing another blast or something else. Looking at him, I realized that he had been injured. Glass had blown in from the window and had cut him on the face. He was bleeding. The three secretaries in the inner office were screaming. I walked over to Mr. Roberts after a minute, helped him up, and walked to the inner office and asked the ladies to help him. I proceeded down the hallway, down the stairs, and to where Post One had been. It was no longer there. It was totally collapsed.

I proceeded back up the staircase to the first floor level. There was a back way out of the Embassy. The key to this back grill gate had been at Post One. I and one of the military men bent the gate and grillwork back as far as we could so that people could crawl out over and climb down the wall at the back of the Chancery into a dirt field. I helped a number of people who had lined up to come out of the Embassy.

I grabbed hold of a young Navy lieutenant who had been in the building, apparently on some business, and told him we had to lock all the safes in the building. We went up to the top floor. Nobody was up there. I said, "As long as we're going through these offices, check and see if there is anybody in here, and secondly, just close the safe and spin the dial."

We checked each floor going into each section. When we got to Communications, there were people shutting down equipment and locking up safes. The thing I remember about the area was that a short distance outside of the vault door, the building had been severed. There was a sheer drop five floors into the concrete. One had to be very careful traversing that part going in.

It was one week to the day that we found the last remains that were found on the site.

One or more people were never found.

There were two distinct occasions after that, and I'm talking about in the next maybe two or three weeks, when I did have a reaction. One was a few nights later in my room in my apartment. Asleep, I found myself startled awake and pushing the blankets off of me very suddenly and sitting upright. I felt I was buried under something. I think, I'm not a psychologist, but I think this is a natural reaction because at the time immediately after the bombing, I recalled meeting with Bob Pugh in front of the Embassy. Bob had basically taken charge and said, "Look, I want you to stay down here on the site and keep in touch with me. I will be down at my apartment where we are setting up. We're in touch with Washington and we need an accounting of people." That was the first real task. An accounting of people. Those who were still missing. Those who were injured. There's no question, Diane Dillard was the focal point for all that. It was apparent right away that there were people who were lost, because there were bodies readily visible. Lebanese rescue people started moving those remains up to American University Hospital to the morgue. We were, and continued for a period of one week, right at the site working with Mr. Hariri's[51] crew and equipment to dig through the rubble, lift up slabs, move them aside, dig, and recover the remains of the victims. I think that in the process of doing that, something was imprinted and later caused me to awake at night and feel as though I was under something and wanted to get out from under it.

The second time was a number of weeks later, and again it was in the apartment. One of the Marines positioned on top of the British Embassy fired at a car which came through a roadblock down on the corniche. It startled me awake and I ended up going down onto the street and talking to the Marines. Fortunately, there was no one hurt. It was a couple of Lebanese men who had been out and had a few drinks and were coming down the corniche and did not see the barbed wire or the roadblock and ran into the wire. The Marine shot at the car.

There was a regional psychiatrist who came in and set up an office, I believe in Diane's apartment, because I recalled going to the Duraffourd building. Everyone had an appointed time to go see the doctor and just sort of talk through how they were doing. At the appointed time I showed up, knocked on the door, and the doctor who was still dealing with the person ahead of me asked if we could reschedule. I said, "Certainly." I had things to do anyway and to be quite honest with you, I never really got back. The Department did the correct things. I think having somebody with professional qualifications come on the scene like that is very helpful. It gives people someone to go to, to cope with that type of trauma.

I guess you deal with it differently at different times. There are some times when it becomes a difficult issue to deal with. It certainly has made me more aware of my own vulnerability in terms of emotional vulnerability. I was a Navy pilot before coming to the State Department and saw a fair amount in terms of aircraft being lost and fellows we went through flight school not surviving. For whatever reason, you moved right along from that. It probably had to be that way in the military, otherwise people wouldn't function so well. This particular event in my life really showed me that you're not quite as tough as you might have envisioned that you were. A lot of wonderful, productive people died that afternoon. Many friends. Acquaintances. That is not easily forgotten. I'm somewhat religious by nature and was brought up a Catholic. I find great confidence or consolation in that. I am perfectly willing to admit that I may be one of these people who are just weak enough in their own selves that they need a crutch to get through life. If that is what it is, I am very comfortable in admitting, religion provides me that. Any one of us could have been a victim. I suppose we would say, "Well, it was God's will that was to be the end of your life that afternoon." And the fact that it wasn't is also God's will.

Keith Quinn, who had been a former supervisor of mine back in the Department, had been sent out to make recommendations with regard to moving to another building. Keith was out there within that first week. I confided in him with regard to a lot of my misgivings. He was very reassuring. I didn't feel terribly effective in Beirut. I don't feel that anyone foresaw the situation being as dangerous as it was. Again, this is with benefit of hindsight. I had had a draft of a cable which was sitting in an in-box the day that we are discussing. Basically, it said that not everything is well, the situation in terms of stability is, we're moving ahead, but there may be an undercurrent, something under the surface. I wasn't sure. I'm not an analyst. No, I didn't see it as terribly, terribly dangerous. I knew that security at the site and in the building was probably not what you might have had at other embassies. There were reasons for that, and certainly the administrative officer and I had discussed that. His views were that we don't want to sink a lot of money into this building because we might not [continue to] be here. We've had to leave it once or twice, and so we're really trying to be reasonable about this. That was his perspective. But looking back, should we have had a perimeter fence around us? Sure, we certainly should have. I recall someone before the blast coming out from Washington and was there specifically to review the security in place. He said, "This is well below any sort of standard that we would have for any U.S. government facility overseas." That was his viewpoint. My view was, give me some money and we'll do whatever we can do with the money we have. At that time, there was no security budget as such. The money wasn't allocated that way. It was regional bureau money or post money that security improvements were made from, and the post understandably did not want to expend a lot of money if it was going to be wasted. [In a March 16 follow-up call, Gannon stated provisions for a fence were made a month before the bombing. "My disappointment was that it was not in October when we settled back in West Beirut rather than in February or March 1983."]

I kept a Beirut file which travelled around with me. I had written a cable back in October of 1982 asking for a review of the security for the Chancery and stating we needed to address this issue now. Basically, that had never really been responded to. I have the cable here in the Beirut file. The cable I'm talking about was dated October 1, 1982. I mentioned that, in my view, now is the appropriate time to dedicate serious effort in installing public access control, which is designed and approved. It's basically a cable asking the Department for assistance. I didn't realize this sentence was in here but, "Hopefully, the problem of vehicle access to the Embassy circular driveway can be resolved as part of the public access control, by installation of a control barrier and an anti-ramming device." This is a cable I wrote and Bob Pugh had signed off on in October and went from Beirut. We never received a response to this cable, but they could always make the argument that, this is October and the bombing took place in April, how many follow-ups did you send?

I found myself dealing increasingly with Bob Pugh and just keeping the administrative officer advised of what we were doing.

I had confidence that Bob was responsive and listening, and the administrative officer was preoccupied with other responsibilities and maybe not focused as much as the DCM was.

When someone goes through something as traumatic as that, you tend to reflect back and ask many questions which have possibly no answers, or at least the answers are not available to us. But, it does have an effect in terms of seeing your own mortality. You see your own vulnerability. You see how easily it can happen. There have been times when I question. Had Dave Roberts not eaten, we would have gone down to get a sandwich and would have been in the cafeteria with you and other people. Virtually everyone except for you and Bob was killed in that room. So I don't think you go through something like that without having some sort of reflection.

To work in the Foreign Service, in and of itself, is not inherently dangerous, but many areas of the world have certain dangers. Being assigned overseas involves a danger not encountered here in Washington. At least you don't have the protection overseas that we have here in the U.S. In many cases you are dealing with people whose grievances against their government or against the U.S. government you could not fully understand. I felt that way with regards to the Middle East. The U.S. lack of success in the world has to do, in my opinion, with a lack of fundamental understanding of what the issues are or what the cultural differences are. We tend to stumble, in some cases, into these situations with the best of intentions, with significant resources, and yet possibly we're missing the whole point of what the problem is. I recall being very frustrated after the incident in Sabra and Shatila, where there were women, children, elderly people murdered by the Phalange. Standing in my office, I said, "I just don't understand how anyone could consider himself a man and look down the barrel of a rifle at a two-year-old and pull that trigger." I felt quite confident that all of humanity would agree with me, only to hear my secretary, for whom I have great regard, say to me, "Mr. Gannon, you don't understand what they've done to us." That was the dawning realization for me that, Dick, you don't understand what the issue is. You don't understand the depth of what has happened in the past.

I guess the Department prepares the Foreign Service personnel as well as they can be prepared for the great unknown. The issue from my standpoint is that people who have joined the Foreign Service must accept the fact that they may be putting themselves, possibly their families, at increased risk simply because they are representing the United States Government abroad. Are they willing to accept that? I think each individual needs to weigh that very carefully, because you do not have the guarantees abroad—even if you are carrying that diplomatic passport—that we basically have here in the States. You don't have the protection. I think the Department has gone a long way in terms of briefing programs, addressing these types of issues, and certainly the Department and Congress have gone a long way in trying to put security resources in the right locales. But then again, terrorism is not something that is easily contained. We no sooner build a secure facility in one country and we have an incident pop up in another country.

The Department has sponsored, with a great deal of effort and money, crisis management exercises for those in Washington and at high-threat posts. It certainly is something that we did not have in Beirut. It's probably a credit to the leadership in Beirut. People really did a magnificent job, I think, given the circumstances and given the fact that they never had any rehearsal. Today many posts have had the opportunity to have a rehearsal, and they should be that much better equipped to address these types of tragedies. Everyone pulled together, pitched in, and did whatever needed to be done at that time. People did what they had to do. You can be assured that people like Diane Dillard, Bob Pugh, and any number of others really performed magnificently in terms of handling a really difficult, difficult situation.

I don't think many of us who were there ever pass by April 18 without pause. You know when it's working up into early April that that is coming. That is always a significant day.

Edited Interview   Barbara Gregory
February 12, 1994   TDY Communications in 1983

I had only been in Beirut for probably five days when this happened. I had lunch with Faith Lee that day. The horrible part of it was that I didn't order the special that day because I didn't like it, so I ordered steak and I got somebody else's. They were slow in the cafeteria. They delivered my steak at the same time as Faith Lee's special, and we finished eating at about ten of one. I stood up and said to Beth Samuel, who was sitting with Dorothy Pech, "All of us get up and get out of here, because we're all too fat and they have a wonderful dessert." It worked out well because if we had not been together, we probably would have had dessert and another glass of wine and we would have been there during the bombing.

I went up to the office and into the back room when everything blew. I thought I was back in Cambodia. I was on my hands and knees trying to get under the equipment because I thought they had zeroed in on us. I thought "Oh, my God, we're going to be hit again with a rocket." I'm on my hands and knees in there, and the door opened and Fred King walked in. All the canisters of tear gas from the fifth floor had exploded and filled up the Communications Center. Faith Lee finally came running in. We didn't have our gas masks. The Marines had taken them all out to check the week before, but had never brought them back. So we covered our faces with paper towels and rushed out. I remember running out into the hall. The sixth floor had this gigantic hole with water running down it. I stopped and was left behind. Everyone else kept running. I just stopped and stared at this and I said, "My God." I remember saying that. I just stood there and I went into total shock.

Then I started down the stairs to get down to the first floor, but there wasn't one. So I came back up and I went down the hall where all the wounded and everybody else had congregated. Beth Samuel was there, bleeding badly. There was a Lebanese woman that had been scalped, and the blood was so thick you could hardly see the tip of her nose. Then the Marines came. A lot of people followed me back to the end of that hall on the second floor. Finally somebody came and smashed in the small window to get to the roof outside. They had us step through the window and out onto the roof, and then we climbed up onto another small roof. They put a barrel up and pushed us up and we got up onto another roof and climbed down a ladder to the back of the Embassy. I remember thinking when I came down, everybody is dead. It was so eerie. It really was. No noise. No nothing. I would come down a few steps and stop and listen. I thought everybody was dead but me. I had forgotten about seeing all my friends running out and thought, "I'm the only one alive." But anyway, it was really traumatic. I went into this shock type thing and I just sort of stayed that way. Then I tried to help out somewhat. We went around to the front of the building, and the police by that time were there. They had guns and said, "Go back." So we all turned around and went back. All I did was feel this horrible, horrible sorrow that somebody could do this to innocent people and their own people. You never get over something like that. It's something I've never gotten over.

I was supposed to have had lunch with Phyliss Faraci the following day. They didn't find her body, I don't think, until, like, Thursday.

I had to go back in three days later, and that distressed me something terribly [sic]; I had to lead the Marines and our people in. They were going up to get the equipment out and they didn't know how to get up there. There was nobody to show them, so I had to go back into the Embassy and climb up to the sixth floor. I could feel the floors shaking. I was very, very nervous about it when I was up there. They were slamming around and I said, "You can't slam around. The only thing holding us up is this pillar." So anyway, I had to lead them back down with some of the equipment and had to return to stay with the remaining equipment and stuff. I stayed there and watched, but it was an awful, awful experience.

State did nothing, absolutely nothing for me. I really, really resented for years and years, well, I still resent, the Department of State's attitude on that. Because I did have friends there. For two days, I thought Diane Dillard had been killed. They gave everyone in the Embassy but me a special R&R back to the States. They said, "Oh, no, you don't get it. You were just here temporary duty." Well, what did that have to do with it? I have never found out.

Then when the psychiatrist came we were supposed to have been informed, but they never told Communications about it. They forgot completely about us.

I was a Rover and left on another assignment, but then they sent me right back into Beirut. Fred King and I were both again stuck in the Embassy when they started bombing the city in August of 1983. We couldn't get out of the Embassy, and the two of us were in the British Embassy though that time. We stayed in the British Embassy. The two of us worked twelve-hour shifts. I never even got a thank you or a job well done. I got nothing out of that. And so we were in the Embassy, like, three days before anybody got in, and then I was there for probably a week and a half after that. Maybe longer. I don't know how long I was there, I can't remember. Mr. Pugh asked me if I wanted to leave, and I said, "I would love to. I don't want to die for Lebanon, I'll tell you." I said, "But I can't, I'm a Rover and I can't just pick up and leave." And he said, "I promise you it won't hurt your career." I went out by helicopter with Carol Madison.

I was in Spain when they blew up the Marines, and I went hysterical in the lobby. And I started screaming, "I'll bet you Reagan's saying it was a dastardly act." That was exactly what he was saying. And I went totally hysterical and I embarrassed myself to the point where I went upstairs and didn't go back out.

It has never, never left me. It has never left. Phyliss I've never forgotten, and I've never forgotten anyone. It's embedded in my brain and I don't usually talk about it. Of course, I don't talk about it to people in Florida. People in Florida don't understand our lifestyle. They really don't. I've told some of them. Once in a while we get into it. It's usually when another Foreign Service person comes that I talk to them. If they haven't been overseas and lived our life, they don't understand it. They think we're showing off. I really don't discuss too much of my life. The Foreign Service was wonderful.

I loved my life. It's just I hated the violence and how it affects me. I was never afraid of thunderstorms or lightning. Now I can't take any loud noises anymore. Thunder makes me so very nervous.

Thunderstorms, that's where I notice it the most, because I used to love them. Now down here, we have the supersonic booms and I practically have a nervous breakdown every time I hear any explosions or loud noises. I don't dwell on it, I just have a hard time with loud explosions, which I never did before, and even in Cambodia they had the rocket attacks. It never really bothered me. But Beirut changed everything. My sister, on our trip to Spain that fall, dropped a window in one of our rooms, and I came tearing out of the bed and my heart was going five million miles an hour. It was just terrible, terrible. It affects everybody. I don't know how anyone could go through something like that and not be affected.

I told [personnel officer] that she can send me any place on earth. I'm willing to go, but I will never go back to Lebanon. I will never go back to Beirut. I will not put myself into that situation. I know it's calm now, but you can send me any place but there. I don't ever want to see it again.

We don't learn lessons. We never have. We have this attitude that everybody really loves us, and they don't love us. Oh, we think we do such good things for them that they really do adore us. Well, they don't. We are so bloody naive and we don't learn lessons. When I went into the Beirut Embassy, I thought, anybody can get in. I wasn't even really thinking about somebody coming in with a truck like that, but I just sat there and thought, we don't have any protection here. We just go merrily along and I don't think we really do learn too much. I mean, the second time they went in. I mean, I'm sorry, but I knew they had moved us into the Embassy on the East side too quickly. We weren't prepared and they could get at us again. We still didn't learn the lesson. It's just like we don't give a darn.

I just found it totally incredible that anybody could do something like this, because they were doing it to their own people. They weren't harming the Americans, because America doesn't care one way or another whether a few of us die, live or die. I like the Arabs and I've always liked the Arabs. They [U.S. officials] sit there and say the Syrians were the ones, but I sit there and say I don't believe it, I think it was the Shiites.

I don't think you can prepare anyone. I really don't. I don't think you can prepare anyone for something like this, do you?

Edited interview 　　　　Faith Lee
January 16, 1994　　　　Communications Officer in 1983

Barbara Gregory and I had just been down in the cafeteria. I had gone back up to my office, because there were two other people who needed to go to lunch. I had just turned to the door to give some messages to Bernard, when the explosion occurred. About 1:05. I said, "What was that?" Bernard had just, like, disappeared. I looked back at the door and he was gone. By that time, the tear gas canisters in the office across from ours had exploded, and tear gas was coming into our office. Of course, we had no other way out except that door. We took wet paper towels and put them up to our face so that we could breathe. That was how we could function, because we had to lock up all the safes and get all the classified stuff together. Then we did get out. I said, "Barbara, make sure you have your purse and passport, because we don't know what has happened." When we got out of the office, we saw that the whole front of the building was gone. When you walked down the hall, the rooms were all gone. It was like walking on a platform on the outside of the building. I thought that we had been RPGed. We had just been hit by one a couple of weeks before, and I thought that this was a super one. I just never thought of a car bomb. Of course, all the elevators were off, so we had to walk down the stairs. We could only get down to about the fourth landing. We saw a lot of people coming out of their offices in various stages of injury. The worse [sic] one I saw was Mary Apovian. She was just covered with blood, because her whole scalp was pulled back.

It was really weird, because no one was screaming or shouting or crying loud. It was like we were all zombies walking down. We got to the second level and couldn't go any further, because the whole front of the building was blown in and we had to get out the back. There was a back window that was over a little shed in the back. There were guys who were working back there. The locals had come over and put a ladder up and helped people down the ladder and go out the back gate. We were all helping each other to get to the ladder. They had to take the ladder away, over to the gate for Mary Apovian, so there was no ladder for us to get down. I think it was about a ten-foot jump. I crouched down and jumped down. I had on sandals and didn't notice until later, when I was walking on the corniche, that my right toe was cut and swollen. I found out I had broken my toe. I wasn't in pain because of the excitement of seeing people injured and trying to get away from the building. The main thing was to get to my apartment to call my family to tell them I was o.k.

When we tried to go to the other side of the Embassy, the Lebanese soldiers there wouldn't let us go through. It was only maybe about 100 yards away to a stairway that led up to a little street. I said, "We just want to go up the stairway." He said tak, tak, tak with the gun. Finally, we walked around the long way through those little cottages behind the Embassy. One of the men, who worked in Administration, lived back there and was serving food to people [who] had not eaten. Barbara and I walked down the corniche. People were talking about a car bomb or a panel truck and that a lot of people had been killed. We couldn't go down around the front of the building, because the French had gotten there first. They wouldn't let us just look. We had to get away.

When I finally got home, I telephoned my mother. It usually took me about 20 minutes to half an hour to get a line for the States. The telephone operator, a friend of mine, had me on line within fifteen minutes. My mother was able to tell my daughter, and about an hour later they had it on the news. People started calling my Mom, and she was able to tell them that I was o.k. This really settled her. People all over knew I was in Beirut, and Mom was able to tell them I was o.k.

I was going on my own R&R because I had planned it about eight months before. I was going to meet my sister the first week in May, this [bombing] happened in April. I was saying to other people that I would have to cancel my trip to meet my sister in Athens. This guy who had come in from Washington said, "Do it. Don't cancel the trip. Do it. You need the trip." So I was able to go and meet my sister for that week and have the cruise, and of course, I felt better afterward.

The bombing made me more alert. It made me more suspicious. When I first came home, I would hear a car backfire, I was, like, jumping, but I got over that. But, it just made me know that you cannot trust, you cannot let your guard down, especially if you're in a post overseas.

You are in such a precarious position, just as the Americans were over there. We should have been walking on eggs over there, but we weren't.

I don't know, maybe we felt invulnerable. I didn't think that anybody was going to hurt me. I wasn't an enemy, so I felt free walking the streets. I never felt threatened. I never felt that they were going to pick me out of a crowd and get me.

My tour ended June 6 of 1983. June 4 of 1983, there was a tremendous earthquake in Beirut that shook the building, my bed. My first thought was, "Oh, shit, the Israelis have struck again." And I ran out on my balcony and looked around. People were down in the courtyard of the building. I asked what it was. They shrugged. Someone came out and said it was an earthquake. I thought o.k., I can deal with an earthquake. I was looking up in the sky for the Israeli planes but saw nothing. So I got ready to go to work. I thought, well, I have two more days, and they're going to bomb me on the 6th of June. *Maasalama* (good-bye).

Now they have support groups to talk to people in bombings and everything. Nothing like that was done. I wasn't injured, so nobody sent me back to Washington to talk to a psychologist or anything. When I went to Japan, a psychologist did come through and said she had been trying to track me down. She came through from Washington and wanted to see me and talk to me. But every time I talked about the bombing and the people I had seen hurt, I would start crying, and even talking to her I would start crying. The one thing I felt within me was to get back to Beirut. I had to get back to see it for myself and see some of the people. She didn't advise it. About three months later, I requested to volunteer to go to Beirut. I went back in May or April of 1984 for TDY. I saw some of the people. I had lunch with Mary Apovian. I met and talked to some of the other people. I was there a month. Now I feel better. This healed me. When I went back to Tokyo, I could talk about the bombing. Now I can talk about it. I don't cry. This was my way of knowing I could be healed.

I think they [State Department] could have followed through on me a little bit more, even though I wasn't injured. I injured my toe, but nothing could be done about that and that wasn't an injury due to the bombing. But I think they could have followed through on me a little bit more. When the Embassy was bombed, I sent a letter asking for help. They didn't have any emergency things for the secretaries to work with. We were running around to the local stores trying to buy pens and paper. I said they should have had an emergency kit of paper, pens, carbons, something like that. He wrote back agreeing. I don't know if they followed through, but they thanked me for that suggestion. I had to go to Hamra Street many times to get paper and pencils and carbon paper. You could hardly find anything. No supplies. They finally started sending in supplies from Washington.

They didn't talk to everybody that was involved in this bombing. No one contacted me. Were they only contacting officers or military people? They should have talked to some of the people that were actually in the building. I don't know why they interviewed a few people that weren't in the building. I had a small camera with me, and I took pictures within the building when I had to go up to my office and make sure I got all of my classified [material] out. But the building wasn't really good for a whole lot of walking and carrying things up and down, but I was responsible. I was responsible for all the classified materials. I was very conscientious about my job but no one contacted me.

You know what I have noticed, when they talk about the bombings? Rarely, rarely do they mention the bombing of the Embassy. They rarely mention the anniversary of our bombing on the 18th of April. They have big things on the big bombing [of the Marines] in October. I feel that the Embassy has been pushed in the corner. There weren't over 200 people killed, but there were a lot of people killed. Maybe it was because a lot of Lebanese were killed and not a lot of Americans. They say, "Oh yeah, it happens." That's it. But the bombing at the Marine barracks, I mean, that's big news. Rarely on the 18th of April do you see anything. They might have a little article in the paper but nothing more.

I feel that somebody knew something and we weren't informed. I read several times that people had been told, but they shoved it off with, "Oh, right, we were going to be bombed." We should have known something was happening, because the French were bombed a week and a half before. But we were so, "Oh, we're the Americans and nobody is going to hurt us." We got too carefree. That's what it was, and we let our guard down. I think we knew something, but we didn't want to admit it. Somebody knew something with all the military people around there, and all "them" around there. They knew something. I guess they figured that we're the Americans and nothing's going to happen to us.

The Embassy was bombed because things were going too well. Every time something went well and the Israelis didn't like it, there would be a bombing. I think I'll go to my death feeling that the Israelis knew something and had a part in it. Because, first of all, where did all those people get all their guns? The Israelis had all the roads blocked and knew everything that was coming and going. They didn't let the Lebanese farmers in with fruit and vegetables. They could have stopped people coming in with guns. I just believe the Israelis knew but they wouldn't tell us. I believe they knew something about the French bombing. They knew. They had infiltrated every place around there.

I don't think the people got who they were trying to get. They killed a lot of Lebanese that were right there at the Consular Section. They didn't get the Ambassador. They didn't get our higher up officers, you know. They got the common people. All the guys in the cafeteria were killed. They got some Americans, mostly military that were down in the cafeteria, but if they had pinpointed certain people, they didn't get them. They wasted Lebanese life.

Well, I tell myself I was warned about Beirut when I was coming into the Foreign Service, I mean, coming into the area. Every situation, I believe, is different. I mean, you might prepare in one way for something and something totally different happens.

Edited interview
November 17, 1993

David H. Mandel
Project Development Officer in 1983

I was in my office, which was on the fourth floor of the building. The way I describe it when people ask me is, I was four floors up and four windows over from the section that collapsed. I had eaten lunch with Kurt Shafer and then went back up to my office. I was reading files when the explosion occurred. I was leaning back in my chair. I had my feet up on the desk and was looking at a file. As a result, my upper body was opposite a column and wasn't opposite the window. If I had been sitting forward, my whole body would have been opposite the window. When the glass flew across I only received cuts, glass cuts to my hands and feet, rather than my face. I was kind of lucky.

I was evacuated out with other people. Some of the military guys got in and let us out. I stood around for a while, not really knowing what to do. Then I walked partway to the street leading up the side hill toward AUH. I walked around there with my hand kind of bleeding all over the place. They grabbed me and put me in an ambulance and drove, much too fast, through town to take me to the hospital. I was dumped out there and was wandering around. A friend who was the Chairman of the Ear, Nose and Throat Department of the hospital found me and took me to his office, where a colleague of his fixed my finger. It was not that serious, my thumb was split and the rest was small cuts. They gave me some shots. It was several hours after the explosion that I wound up in his office, and things were already starting to calm down.

At the time the Embassy was blown up, Malcolm Butler, who was the Mission Director, was away in the States. Bill McIntyre, who was the Deputy, was killed. As the third most senior officer, I got a battlefield promotion to Acting Mission Director. As soon as I was patched up, I felt they were counting on me to be the one to find out where everybody was and what was happening, to get the things together, to be the contact point, clear out the stuff, and re-establish the office in an apartment. We got an empty apartment in the Duraffourd and so we began getting our files together. As I recall, two or three days after the explosion, we had a meeting with an engineering firm which had scheduled a visit sometime earlier. We were functioning and back in business after a couple of days. I was just really busy with that. You don't stop and think about things. You just keep going.

My wife and I were very lucky. Under normal circumstances, we would have been eating in the cafeteria. Because that particular day Jill chose to go shopping, I went down to eat early and went up early.

Two psychiatrists came to provide some assistance to people. I was too busy and personally didn't participate. The woman psychiatrist, Christine Bieniek, got the wives and ladies together. I think it was very voluntary, sort of: "They are here. If you need them, you can come." I was very busy, and I told everybody Malcolm said that when he came back he was going to go and talk to her to kind of lead the way, but I don't think a lot of people did go. This was ten years ago and we were learning a lot of things at that time. I don't think that the people in the business really understood all of the ramifications. I don't think the State Department at that stage was all that sensitive and concerned. I mean they were, "Just get on with the business and if you need help, it's there." It's not like now: when you get some sort of really traumatic experience, they send in whole teams. They have organized activities and they say, everybody will come and we'll talk. It's much more aggressive, because people like me are very introspective. My tendency is to withdraw into myself. Far as I know I did fine. I didn't have any real problems, but I think there are people who draw into themselves and do have problems, and unless the assistance that is being offered is more pro-active, it sometimes doesn't reach the people it needs to reach. Beirut was the first time that we and the United States Government facilities were really subjected to this kind of stuff outside the military. It was the early days. My impression is that now when things like this happen, State is a lot more pro-active in going after people and saying, "Wait a minute, wait a minute, sit down and let's talk."

That Security Overseas Seminar has been improving over the years. I took it six or seven years ago, and I think they do a pretty good job of briefing people. I saw a film about coping with the terrorists' acts, and there is one with a clip of me in it. I was very angry about it, because they never talked to me about it. I got very angry when they were carting me away in the ambulance and someone stuck a T.V.

camera in the ambulance. I had not had a chance to contact my kids, and I was afraid it would turn up on T.V. before I talked to them and they would really get upset. I got really angry with the guy poking the camera in my face, and they kept that as a background clip in one of these films. They did it without my permission and I was very upset.

Since I've been in Beirut, I find that most missions overseas base their briefing of new people on the current level of threats. Everybody's perception is that the post is real safe. They don't really worry about emergency evacuation plans or what. I think that's a mistake, because things can change pretty quickly and if people aren't prepared before, then you run into problems. I think there needs to be a greater emphasis in overseas missions. In Washington, they have this course and they think it is fine. When you get to post, emergency evacuation plans, bomb preparedness plans, who's responsible for what, that sort of stuff, should be run through with people. But it isn't done. They are supposed to be briefing the newcomers but it doesn't take place. People tend to avoid. It's a real problem.

They say, it can't happen here. It's very safe. A safe post tends to get a little sloppy, and it's hard to get people to keep their guards up. I tend to say the people who have experienced the full consequences of not keeping their guard up are more inclined to take precautions.

I still sense that my kids are very upset about the whole thing. The biggest problem was notification. They were all in boarding school. One way or another, most of them found out about it through the news. All they heard was that the Embassy was blown up. They had to wait several hours before they found out whether we were safe or not. It was very hard on them, particularly our younger son, who at the time was twelve or thirteen. I think they still have vivid recollections and a lot of anger about [it]. There isn't much you can do, but I think that there's got to be a better way. I know the problem is striking the balance between calling and saying we don't know or we are waiting for information, and wanting to be sure that the information is right so that you don't notify somebody that somebody's o.k., and it turns out they are dead or that they are hurt. But it took a long time before there was any notification. I think that most of the notification came through our friends we called four or five hours after the bombing.

I don't think the Department did anything about notifying my kids and the schools that they were in. I don't think they handled it very well. My youngest son was quickly palmed off on his godmother, who lived near the school, and she had to cope with it. The other kids, I don't think they really, really knew what to do. An awful lot of Foreign Service children go to boarding school. It seems to me that something could be done about that. No one thought about the kids. Let's put it this way, if there was anything available, we were unaware of it. I know that they have counseling services, but you have to go find it. Nothing was offered to us as far as I know.

The bombing is a distant memory. I don't think about it very much any more. It's hard for me. I'm not very introspective, so I don't know what to say about how I feel about it. I mean, obviously, I have all the same feelings now I had then. It probably shouldn't have happened. We should have been more careful. I guess the long-term effect on me personally is that I'm very security-conscious. I tend to be the one to keep my guard up. When I went to Oman, our offices were just apartments. My office looked right out on the parking lot, and it was a first floor office with windows opened right on an area where all kinds of people parked. It made me very nervous, obviously. By the time we moved, our building finally met security standards. As a senior management mission manager, I'm involved with Emergency Action Committee. I tend to be the one who argues with keeping the guard up, because you never know when the situation can change. I'm quite a bit more security-conscious than people who have not been through the Beirut bombing.

Obviously there is cocktail talk. We get together and people ask about my experiences, and when they find out that you've been in Beirut, they ask me to tell them about it and we go through all the physical stuff, what happened and all that. We don't really talk about it much.

I don't think it changed my life in any major way. We stayed on. We kept working.

Our careers followed a normal pattern. I don't think it's had any dramatic effect.

Actually, it was kind of interesting; with the ten-year anniversary they held that memorial service for the Marines. I said, "Gee, fine. Think about it for the Marines, but nobody thought about it for all those people that died in the Embassy." At least, I never saw anything like a memorial service like they did for the Marines.

It really is funny how the whole institutional memory seems to suppress that, the whole remembrance of it. I think it's part of the cycle of, "Oh God, look what happened. We've got to spend money, spend money." But now, all of a sudden we're starting to get this, "Boy, why are we spending all this money on security? Look at this waste of money."

We're on a downswing and have been for several years, with budget cuts and deficits. How do we justify this and that? I get really nervous when I see that kind of thing happening. That really bothers me. People forget, and all of a sudden you go from one extreme to the other. Of course, right after, we had the Inman Commission,[52] and all our embassies were fortified and reinforced.

Edited interview
December 11, 1993

Dorothy Pascoe
Secretary to Ambassador in 1983

It didn't really affect me all that much, I don't know if I'm a strong personality or what. I was crushed that so many people and friends were killed, but personally, it didn't bother me. It really didn't. We had the psychiatrist there, and I didn't need to talk to her because I didn't <u>need</u> to. I don't know if I'm some sort of a weird person or what. I really felt so bad for the young Marine downstairs, and for our social secretary who had just gotten downstairs, and all the people in Consular Section. I was worried sick about Dorothy Pech, because she had been down in the Administration Section getting money changed and I just knew it hit there.

I was on the eighth [floor] in the office with the Ambassador and the DCM and the Administrative Officer. I was just sitting there, because I was waiting for Dorothy to come back so that I could go to lunch. The Ambassador was getting all ready to go out for his run at the school. He always did the laps. A phone call came in for him. I was sitting with my back to the windows. It was kind of a rainy day, cloudy, and we had some thunder. So when it hit, I thought it was a clap of thunder. Then I remember seeing this bright light out of my right eye and I thought, "No, I think something has hit this building." People do funny things. I ran to the little room where we kept our coffeemaker. I stood in the doorway, like you do in an earthquake. It was really strange and I said, "Dorothy, this is not an earthquake." I screamed for the Ambassador and ran into his office. I was trying to lift the flagstaff off the Ambassador when the DCM and the administrative officer came tearing in. We pulled it off and ran over to the window to look outside towards the University side.

We saw all the kids standing along the fence there. We couldn't see down. The eighth floor sat back and the front was sheared off. It was even. By that time, we were starting to smell the stuff from the bomb, and we decided we'd better get the heck out. I said, "Well, there is a window in the Ambassador's bathroom." So we ran out that way because it got us out on a roof, and then there were steps that took us up a little higher. By that time, the Ambassador's security guards came tearing up the steps looking for him, and we all walked down the steps and checked all the floors as we went down. The Marines were checking out all the floors and there was nobody else on the floors. I think it was the second or third floor that we crawled out a window, and then down and around the back porch on the corniche side, and up another ladder and over a wall. The Ambassador went one way towards the corniche, but they wouldn't let me go that way. I had to go another towards the back. We all just kind of stood around, not really knowing what to do. You really wanted to help, but they wouldn't let us help. In fact, I went around the other side toward like the front of the building. I can't remember if it was the French there, it wasn't our Marines, but there were some people there with guns, and they wouldn't let us go towards them. So, at that stage of the game I wondered, what does one do. I thought that the best thing for me to do would be to go back to the apartment and wait to hear from someone. I just waited for a while, and then I started calling around but couldn't reach anyone. Finally, Dorothy Pech called me and said they were having a meeting down at the DCM's apartment. I really lit into Pugh when I found that out. I really let him have it both barrels when I got to his place. Here I am the Ambassador's secretary, and nobody was calling me. I was really ticked off.

I guess not a heck of a lot went through my mind really. I kind of didn't even give it a thought at the time. Of course, you wonder afterwards why something like that happens, but over there you don't have to wonder why anything happens. Things just happened all the time for no damned reason at all. Car bombings. We used to look out the window and see blow-ups on the corniche. The Ambassador and I sat there at the window and saw a car just blow right up. Nothing really went through my mind at that time. I wasn't scared. I just couldn't believe it. A lot of people were kind of in shock.

Later on, I got a little bit leery because of where I lived. I used to see the guy who ran our apartment building do some strange things. A car stopped right out front once and they pulled some guy over, beat the heck out of him, threw him in the car. All kinds of strange things were going on around there at that time.

I don't think I was frightened at all. I really, honestly, to this day, I don't think I was ever frightened. I think I was more excited, the old adrenaline starts pumping away. I know it was horrible, but I certainly wasn't scared. I was really more excited about, "My God, what's going to happen next." I was more frightened when we were evacuated at the Ambassador's residence. Because those RPGs were coming around the Ambassador's so much. We used to go outside and stand on the patio and watch everything that was going on. It was horrible. Well, the residence did get hit in a couple of places, but not badly. I really was a little more frightened then, than after the bombing after the Embassy.

I was wondering what to do, because I would have really liked to go and help. I did go as soon as we were allowed. I went to the hospital and visited.

A lady psychiatrist came out and talked to a lot of the people. I just didn't talk to her. I just didn't feel I needed it, and it's really never bothered me since then. The thought of all my friends, you know, the people that I knew, getting killed and the other ones getting injured, that was about the worst thing, but it didn't seem to affect me personally. It's weird.

The bombing was just plain craziness, that's all. Why would people do that? It was probably one of those strange little factions there that really had it in for the Americans. I'm sure there were quite a few of the groups that were very, very anti-American there. Maybe for being on the side of the Israelis during that time, earlier on.

The bombing didn't make any difference in my life. I look back, of course. Many people ask, "Oh, you were in Beirut, were you there during the bombing?" I have to go through this whole thing with them, where I was, how I felt and the whole thing. It's about the only time I really think about it. I mean, I remember that I was there and what happened. Sure, I think about it. Not in a bad way, because I tell everybody that I really enjoyed my tour while I was over there and I did! I really did enjoy my tour with everything that was going on. When you go into the Foreign Service, as far as I'm concerned, you've got to expect something like this. Particularly in these volatile type countries. When I first arrived, my God, the militia was on every corner. You just kind of got used to that. But even with all of that going on, we could still get around. I used to go get my hair done, go up to the market, and you know, no problem, until this happened.

I had been in Taiwan when the students rioted there and we closed the Embassy there. It was kind of out of the blue. We were all getting ready to leave, and POW. We couldn't leave because the Embassy was surrounded, and I found it <u>very</u> exciting. I'm weird, I'm telling you, I'm weird. Things don't seem to scare me. They kind of excite me. Because I thought, boy, I've heard about these things and now it's happening to me.

I just never gave it a thought, that my life was in danger. Particularly in Beirut, I just never really thought about it. Gosh, after we got down and worked at the British Embassy, heck, I was running a sorority in my apartment. I must have had eight girls there. They did not want the girls staying so far off. Every bed was full. The couches were full.

We had to be very careful while we were in the British Embassy. The lack of water, the lack of electricity, and that kind of stuff gets to you more than anything else.

When I was in Israel in late 1973, the Syrians bombed. I was on the eleventh floor in this little room. I said, "Well, if I'm going to get bombed, I think I'd rather be on the ground." I think [I] was more scared then than I've ever been really.

And then we had the kidnapping down in Santo Domingo. I just kind of got prepared for these little things. You know, none of this ever really bothered me. Like I said, I think I was most scared sitting up there in that little room during that air raid, which didn't last anytime at all.

I cannot remember ever hearing instructions on what might happen and what one should do to prepare yourself. But I think it might be a good idea. I think that's why they're not getting so many people in the Foreign Service any more and why so many secretaries are getting out.

I've thoroughly enjoyed my Foreign Service life. I really did. I liked all the places, I wish I could have gone to other places and, but [sic] I really enjoyed all of my posts, every one of them.

Edited interview　　　　　Dorothy Pech
January 11, 1994　　　　　Secretary to Deputy Chief of Mission

    I had been married in Beirut, many moons before in the late fifties, and returned when our first son was nine months old. My husband's family was from there. So, you see, I knew Beirut in the old days. Our home was a very simple apartment, a small building. Actually, the apartment was quite big. It was in Beirut, the green line area where the movie district used to be. In 82/83 before the Embassy bombing, I walked down in there and I actually found the apartment. The 82/83 winter was when things were getting better in Beirut. The glass was being cleaned up in the green line. Lights were going up in the old section of town. The funny thing I remember on that famous day, as we were all eating lunch, was the Administrative Officer saying how things were getting so much better that surely our differential would go down. Who would have guessed that a few minutes later... We were sitting in the middle of the cafeteria. I even remember what I ate that day, that famous lemon sauce with rice. There was Beth Samuel and myself. Tom Barron and Lisa Piascik came over to the table. Beth was always on a diet but wanted to stay and have some dessert. I said, "No, Beth, no dessert. We have to go, besides I have to cash a check. Come on, it's almost 1:00, we have to go." So I made everybody leave. I got up to the cashier's over on the other side and just had finished the check when everything just fell down. I fell down, but I didn't know what hit me. It must have been a piece of the ceiling or some wall. I was cut across my forehead but was able to walk. I bled a lot. They later found my check still in the book, by the way. It just happened. You didn't know if it was an earthquake or a bomb from the sky. It was just so fast and unexpected. Especially when things were getting so much better. How to get out of the place? You can't get out. That was one of our biggest things. Seriously injured people, trying to get them out. We were up on the third floor and most people were fairly calm, but we simply couldn't find a way. Someone from the Red Cross finally came in and said, "Come on, you at the end." Because I looked like I'd lost my eyes. I kept saying, let the really injured go. Then we had to go down the stairs and jump quite a ways, maybe about three feet or something like that, to another building. There was a Marine on the other side. I said, "I can't do it," but he said, "You have to do it." So I did it and he grabbed my hand. Then I was able to go down a ladder, just sort of dripping as I went. Then they threw me in a car. I was alone and going by with just the one eye and seeing the devastation, the person that was hanging. At the hospital, the main idea was to take care of the seriously injured, naturally. That was like a MASH operation. We were all lying all over on benches, watching those go through who were serious. Eventually the doctor came and just said, "Lie very still. You were very lucky. Just a breath more..." Without anything, they sewed up several stitches in that big main room. There were a bunch of us. Beth was there with a lot of glass, but again, we could walk and talk, so they had to take care of the others first. It was very calm. I'm usually calm in a crisis. Some people react differently, you know, scream and holler. It wasn't until we had gone to the hospital that we started filtering through what had happened. We were just mostly concerned about others and glad we could walk. Other people started to tell us what had happened, you know how it filters through the grapevine.

The main thing was, I don't know how long I was at the hospital. I can't remember, but I was taken home by Tish Butler, who lived across the hall from me in that nice building, and the AID secretary Rikkie Smith. It was the first time I could not be alone, I must admit, and I am usually fiercely independent. I called Bob Pugh and said, I can't be alone. That is very rare for me, but I just couldn't. I went to his apartment and proceeded to stay just a few days to help. I only could see with one eye. I stayed a few days and then eventually I went back. So I have often said that in my opinion, it is wise not to be left alone and that people need to work. It helps even if you can only hobble or are one-eyed. There is something about it, and I think this was true of most everyone. It's the time that [sic] when you don't want to be the cat that licks its wounds. You just needed other people around and to work and feel useful and do something.

Then I was able to stay alone at night, but generally I kept busy and worked and tried to go out with friends. I just didn't like the aloneness thing. Then they wanted some of us to leave on R&R and very much wanted me to do that, and I didn't want to. I was due home leave. I wanted to go on leave because my son was graduating from college, but I wanted to come back. I feel it was the best thing for me.

It was absolutely the best psychological therapy. Mind you, I'm pretty tough.

It wasn't until six weeks later when I was home and I went down to Texas, where my son was graduating from college, when he and I were out in a little courtyard with a glass of champagne, that I started to tell him about something. I barely could talk and I felt so stupid, but the tears started coming. It was the first time I'd done it and it was probably good for me. So, then I'm able to talk about it. I think that is good. Everybody thought that I was crazy to return to Beirut, but I'm very glad I did.

Beirut was an experience in my life. Of course, I didn't have a spouse that died or something. No, I think about it once in a while. I learned how fast something could happen. You know, the talk of the differential being cut. It's just what blows your mind. I mean, I can remember that so vividly...thinking that my life [was] over with.

I don't know if you want to call it fate or what not, but I don't believe much in anything like that, but in a way had I been in the cafeteria, in the elevator, at my desk... I had just finished my check and looked at my watch and said, "Oh, damn, it's five after one, I'm late...I have to get back." That's when, of course, it went off. But, had I been at my desk—the beautiful picture window that was behind me managed to come all over my desk and I just would have been...[makes cutting noise].

The Department sent out some psychiatrists, psychologists, or whatever. They came even while I was at Bob Pugh's, within a few days afterwards, but I chose not to talk to them. I suppose they must have thought, Oh! she's one of those. I was handling this myself. I didn't have anything to say. I had to work through it. I was fine. It worked out. I worked through by working and talking to friends. What should I do, come back here? Who would understand anything like that? To me, what helps are colleagues who understand. Family, but what do they know? They couldn't possibly understand, except to moan and groan and feel sorry and say, why do you go to these crazy places. But, for me that was the key. I don't think it changed my life. I'm very much Foreign Service, I like it.

I always smile when all these security people come around, because I say, "Just tell me how many ways I can get out of a building. Don't give me one front door." It's ludicrous, and you have all these emergency actions. One thing. I just try to keep a little cool about it. We were very lucky. I thought Bob Pugh did marvelously in being cool. The security person, Dick Gannon, was very cool and calm and that helps a lot. Diane Dillard went about her business setting up her household, and what more could the department do? I think that they are very good in a crisis to try to help us. Some of us just don't want to be pushed, and just leave us be. I talked more. Talking helps. Talk with colleagues, people who can understand. It's no good with others. What is a psychiatrist? I don't care if he has twenty degrees, you feel sort of silly...like what does he understand; it's got to be your colleagues.

I don't like to talk to them [Foreign Service psychiatrists] too much.

I think of the tragedy of that young gal who was on TDY, Deborah Hixon. I had taken her to lunch the day before. I think about these sort of things. She was talking about how there were two children, she and her brother. Her brother had died in a tragedy, a car accident or some sort of accident. He was, like, 19 and her parents have never gotten over it. So, we are sitting there talking, I liked her and she loved to do this sort of thing. I think that was a little hard. We went through some of her things. That was a bit difficult. I get a bit choked on that, because she was about 28. I was going to go back and talk to her parents, and also to Bob McMaugh's, the Marine. I had talked to him that morning, too. He said he wasn't feeling well and I jokingly said, "Oh, well, maybe it will be a short day." The things like that I pondered a long time, and you remember these things. Fifty years later, you remember these things, it's not funny but...I did chat with him. I did get very broken up. Beth and I did, when the Marine was brought through. We were out to the airport when they sent them back. That was hard, I was choked hard with that. Again, you just work it through. I don't have a lot of suggestions other than to each his own.

Edited interview　　　　　　Daniel J. Pellegrino
January 14, 1994　　　　　　Defense Attaché's Office in 1983

    I was sitting right at my desk. I had to make a phone call, and as soon as I picked up the phone, I didn't even have a chance to dial the number, the bomb went off. When I saw all the damage in my office, everything was dangling from the ceiling, and all the smoke and dirt, I thought my office took a direct hit [from] the RPG's. I thought that somehow somebody knew that I was working in intelligence, and they just put something right into my office. So then I said to myself, wait a minute, maybe that's only the first round, maybe there's a dozen more on the way. I didn't want to make any quick moves, because I remembered from my time in Viet Nam they had instructed us that if you're getting a mortar barrage or a rocket barrage, you don't want to panic and start running wildly, because there might be a dozen more rounds coming in and you could end up dead if you make the wrong move. So I didn't want to rush out of the room right away. Then I began thinking how big it was, because I had been sitting at my chair and then the next thing I knew I was standing. It actually brought me out of the chair. It was awful big and loud. I thought for a second—because you know how the Israelis had come in and bombed—that maybe they had made a mistake and bombed the Embassy by mistake. But they wouldn't have done that, because they were known for using the precision weapons, so I don't think they would have made that mistake. Then I thought, maybe the Syrians had bombed us, and then I put that out of my mind. Then I started looking around and started hearing Sally Johnson screaming. I thought, "Whoa." The way she was carrying on, the other side of the office must have gotten hit, too. The way she was carrying on, I thought maybe she was dying. I told myself that if I look around and see the wall behind me, I would be o.k., but if the wall was not there, I was probably going to be hurt. I couldn't feel anything at all. My ears were ringing, whistling, so I put my hands up to my head to see if the top of my head was there, my ears were there. The only thing I felt was like this little burning on my back. I took my hands down and they were full of blood, and I couldn't figure out where it was coming from because I didn't feel anything. All of this blood was all over the front of my shirt. I said, gee, and then started swearing. I knew this was going to cause a lot of problems. My family is going to be worried. I kept thinking, should I make a move because they had told us to get to the middle of the Embassy if anything happened. I was waiting and waiting and waiting trying to figure out what I should do, the next move I should make. Then I saw, I think I saw, Colonel Craig leave. Then Major Englehardt came in, looked at me and said, "Well, you're not too bad." Later I started smelling the tear gas, and one of the Marines came in with his gas mask on and he gave me a little medical patch to put on my head. I remember carrying one of those things for three years when I was in the Army, and I carried one every day in Viet Nam and never had to use it, and here I am in Beirut and here is a Marine giving me his medical packing to put on my head. I made my way through the office and saw all the damage, and they were just carrying Sally Johnson out. She was hurt pretty bad in the head. I got into another room on the other side of the hall. I asked Colonel Craig for a towel, because I felt like I needed to blow my nose. I blew my nose and the towel just came out full of blood. So we were just there, we really didn't know what to think or what to do. I decided to go out and take a look to see if it was safe. One of the Lebanese who worked in the Embassy motioned to us to come along. I remember turning around and looking out where the wall used to be and looking out into the Mediterranean Sea. There was just rubble below and then the sea. Then it really hit me that we got hit by something really massive. It couldn't have been an RPG, because the damage was so massive. I got down to the fourth floor and then I saw all the other people: the McCulloughs, Dorothy Pech, and Dick Gannon. There was this large beam that came right up through the window, and Dick was trying to push it out of the way so we could possibly climb out the window. It wouldn't budge. Everyone I saw was bleeding. Someone motioned us to come down the other stairwell. Again, I was real apprehensive, because I didn't know how much damage had been done. We finally got down to the second or third floor and they led us to a window and down the ladder. When I got down, I saw there was an ambulance, so I got in and took off with that wailing siren. Traffic was bumper-to-bumper, inching along and stopping. The Lebanese came up and peered at me. It was unsettling. When we got to the hospital, the nurses were waiting for me and led me into a part of the room where they had set up the seriously wounded and the less wounded. Just as I came in, I heard something behind me and I turned around. They had brought somebody in on a sheet. It was a body, and there was nothing but hamburger. They put me in a room with all these people that were hurt. I can remember just sitting there and bleeding. Finally, a doctor came in and said that everybody had to get two tetanus shots. Those hurt. Then I started hurting all over, from the top of my head. My hand started throbbing. I started seeing where the blood was coming from. They came over to me and cut my shirt off. It was one of my favorite shirts, and they cut it off and I asked if my back was okay. They started cleaning it. It was filled with little tiny shards of glass that somehow had gotten down my shirt and was [sic] scratching me. It didn't draw any real blood, but it was irritating. They started working on me and cleaning me, and started stitching me, and they had to go into my hand with a pair of long tweezers to pull out glass. They had to sew up my scalp and my neck and my face. The nurse came behind me and held my head while the needle was going in, 'cause I kept pushing my head back. She was pushing forward, and the needle was going in and made me wince every time they did it. Finally they had me patched up, and I saw a young Lebanese man come in. His arm looked like a biology book which explains how you have the top layer of skin, and the next layer, and the next layer. He must have been in shock. His arm was opened up and they directed him to go some other place.

I had to buy some antibiotics and I didn't have enough Lebanese money on me. In fact I didn't have any money on me, so I had to borrow from Diane Dillard to pay for these antibiotics. Colonel Craig showed up. He had commandeered a Marine driver and jeep and drove me to his apartment.

Colonel Craig said to be in the next morning at 8:30. The normal time was 7:30; I think we came in an hour later or something and that was it. I think a couple of days off right then and there would have been time to fall back and regroup and recharge your batteries for a couple of days. Give yourself time to compose yourself and let you start thinking. Any kind of traumatic thing takes a couple of days and then, you know, you see how you feel.

I remember we were down at the airport when they brought the seventeen caskets out, and a lot of the Americans were crying, and all of a sudden, a colonel said, "Well, everybody was a volunteer." It sort of made sense to me. Nobody's arm was twisted to go there. Everybody knew there was a risk there, and I knew what it was like to be in a war zone. Although it was unexpected when the bomb went off, it was always in the back of my mind that something like that could happen.

The State Department people brought in one or two medical doctors and at least one psychiatrist. All they did was say, "Well, if you want to, if you feel you need to see the psychiatrist, you can see him." I had been to Viet Nam and we had gotten mortared and rocketed many nights, and I didn't feel I needed to see him. I felt I got off kind of lucky compared to the other people, compared to that person they brought in behind me at the hospital.

I knew that the threat was going to go from the Embassy to individual Americans, but I don't know how much extra security they were providing for the people, and at times I felt personally threatened.

Somebody decided that everybody had to take their bandages off. They wanted the people to take their bandages off. They didn't order you to, but they said, "We would like to have the people take their bandages off." They want to make it look like there weren't that many people hurt, or something. I remember the pictures of John Reid. He did take a lot of his bandages off, because when I first saw him he was wrapped up like a mummy, and then he took some of them off and I guess they only left on the ones that were absolutely necessary.

I took my R&R the last part of May; early June [I] called Bobby McMaugh's father on the phone. He broke down on me, and I'm not really good at those kinds of things and I really didn't know what to say, but when he broke down, it was really tough. This last time [in Washington, D.C.] I saw him in person, and we talked for a good two hours or more. He still has a lot of anger, a lot of anger.

I think the Embassy was bombed due to negligence of some people who didn't think it could really happen. The American Embassy was sort of sacred, and they thought it would never get bombed. A lot of people didn't think the threat to Americans was really there. I think there was negligence. Beirut was a free-fire zone in those days, and they should have known that we really needed to beef the security up. I can remember my first month there, they shot Major Hoff and then shortly after that, they had put some sort of explosive up against the wall one night. I asked right then and there, why didn't we move to east Beirut. Why couldn't we just get out of here and go to the east side where it was safer? Someone said we couldn't do that, because it would look like we're taking sides and abandoning west Beirut.

We were trying to force negotiations on the Syrians, and these militia groups were getting bolder and bolder. They thought they could do something like that to scare all the Americans out, and they do have terrorists who just like to commit terrorist acts for themselves, not for any political reasons. There were so many different groups over there, it could have been one of those that actually carried out the bombing just for the sake of carrying it out. They wanted Lebanon to be divided and they didn't want to have peace. Americans were trying to bring peace of some sort with negotiations, et cetera. They felt that by lashing out, they could keep things unstable there.

What bothered me was that people [Americans] didn't seem to be real concerned about safety. They could have beefed up a little bit more on personal security.

I've heard from a knowledgeable source that they were trying to get the CIA people.

But then I also heard that they were trying to [get] Habib and Draper and the Ambassador.

Later when I was in Korea, a State Department team gave a one-day training seminar on terrorism for intelligence and law enforcement people. It was just pictures of actual scenarios or actual terrorist acts. They told how these terrorists act. That was a real eye-opener. I think they should do something like that [for] FSOs. Later, when I started at Attaché School there at Anacostia, the instructor came in the first day and said, "Well, here is your first class and it's about terrorism, and the first thing I want to tell you is that if somebody's out to get you, they're going to get you. They wanted the American Embassy in Beirut and they got it. They wanted the Marines and they got them." So if you're forearmed with this knowledge of how these people act and their objectives and goals and how they go about it, you have an understanding. At least the United States government should arm you with that before they send you someplace.

It's something that you never forget and I broke that rule they told us about in Viet Nam. About not ever getting close to anybody; don't become good buddies. I did that with McMaugh. He was the one at Post One.

I think about it from time to time. They just had the tenth year anniversary of the Marine bombing on T.V. They talked about the Middle East and Lebanon and Israel. I always keep track of terrorism. I'm always interested. I'm always looking. I'm always down at the bookstores and the library. I always manage to wend my way over to the biography section and the current events, and always have my eye [open] about that period of time and there have been a number of books written.

Edited interview   Beth Samuel
February 12, 1994   USIS Secretary in 1983

In 1982 I was in personnel in Washington and couldn't get anybody to go to Beirut. I was making assignments for secretaries. Two people bailed out within about two months, because their families put so much pressure on them. I called John Reid and Joan Sallis in Beirut. Both said there was stuff going on but basically it was o.k. So my husband and I decided to go. I had to actually push my agency to let me go. They tried to talk me out of it but I persisted.

On April 18 I had just left the cafeteria. I've said many times that being fat saved me, because I'd gone on a diet that Monday. I was so hungry that I went to lunch about 20 minutes early and left the cafeteria at 1:00. The bomb went off at 1:06. Normally I would have been there. I was standing at my desk sorting through the cables, and the next thing I knew, I was on the floor. Lots of cuts, because we were on the front, facing the corniche. There was lots of glass and boards falling from the walls. I was knocked to the floor and came to, and there I was with everything sticking to me. Blood everywhere, but I walked out under my own steam. It was so strange, because I never thought the bomb was in our building. I heard a whoosh—a little wind, and I thought, boy, that was close. The next thing I knew I woke up and was on the floor. I knew what had happened but didn't have time to think about it. I just thought it was nearby. It never occurred to me that it would be us. Never; that was naive wasn't it?

There was lots of smoke. I guess I didn't really think it was a bomb. I just knew there was debris everywhere and people were screaming and crying. John Reid's desk went down the hole. He was sitting at the desk when it happened and was blown forward. Neither one of us thought about how close we came until we went back up there about five or six days later to see what we could salvage in the way of equipment, and we realized that his desk was gone. I saw the smoke and everything coming out of John's office, and I went in there to see about him, hollering, "John, John, are you all right?" He said, "No, I'm not," but I couldn't see anything, because it was all smokey. He was lying on the floor and his legs were pinned down by a piece of wood. The walls had fallen in, obviously. He got out and came walking over to me. Two of the military guys came in and took us out and sat us down in the hall. They figured we were all in shock, which we were, I'm sure. We just kind of sat there until the security people came up to take us out, to lead us outside. They wanted to be sure there were no more bombs around. The next thing I remember was being taken out the back door toward a wire fence. The people up there lifted us over to the ambulances. We got to the gate and the damned thing was padlocked. They couldn't get it unlocked. It had rusted shut. Here were all these injured people standing there bleeding, and we couldn't get out the back gate. It's funny now, but it wasn't funny then. I remember these Marines came by and said, "Shoot the mother----er." They finally got it. I learned later that this was just one of the glitches. You know that the Marines would practice raids at night. They would have to go out in the middle of the night and pretend that a strike had taken place. They had told GSO about that gate. They couldn't get it open. The lock needed to be sawed off and nothing had been done about it. So they lifted us over. To this day I don't remember Dennis Foster, but he says that he helped lift me over the fence to the ambulance. I was just totally in shock, because even now I don't remember it.

A friend, Annalisa Meyer, saw the bombing and ran down the Corniche to find out what was going on and ran into Kurt Shafer who told her that I was injured but walking.

Bless her, she called my mother. She saved my parents a tremendous amount of trauma by telling them before they saw it on T.V. My husband was driving to work and heard [it] on the radio.

Bob Pugh had a meeting at 8:30 the next morning, and it never occurred to anyone not to go. I don't think it occurred to anybody not to get up and go to work. You felt better being there. That's what I remember. It felt good being with other people that had been through it, and you didn't want to be with anybody else. And John and I talked about this. I talked to the psychiatrist about it, too. I said the only thing that I feel a little bit guilty about is that I don't have any desire to be home or to talk to my family or to talk to my husband. I feel that these [colleagues] are the people I want to be with right now. They told me that was very normal.

They brought in two psychiatrists, one from Cairo and one from somewhere else. But we all thought it was just a big farce, and we kind of hooted about it later. Somebody said, "I think they learned a lot talking to us." By the time they brought them in, it was too late. We had all done our crying. We had had each other as therapy. That's what everyone talked about for days and days.

John and I both looked awful, but we healed quickly. We had a lot of cuts on our faces, but they were just surface cuts and we didn't look bad for a long time. About three weeks later, the desk officer in Washington wanted us both to leave on R&R. I said, let John go first because he needs it worse than I do. He was the one that had to identify the bodies of the three USIS employees who were killed. It really upset him. In June I went home for three weeks. It never occurred to me not to go back. That's what sounds so strange, I guess. In Washington, people would say, "Oh, where are you going next?," and I said I hadn't thought about it because I had to go back to Beirut. They were just astonished that I was going back to Beirut. I hadn't even thought about it until they questioned it, because my tour wasn't over, so obviously I was going back. I guess that was the old Foreign Service pro. It just never occurred to me not to go back. So I went back to Beirut, and I stayed there until the end of October in 1983. They were already taking people out. Carol Madison, the Assistant PAO, got evacuated. It was just a matter of time before I would have been evacuated, too, so I left at the end of October.

I don't think there is any sense to be made of it. To me, the whole Middle East doesn't make sense the way they fight. There is so much hatred in everybody's mind and they instill it in their own children. It just keeps going on, generation after generation. The revenge—well, your grandfather shot my father so I'm going to shoot you. This kind of thing and I don't think it makes any sense. I don't think there is any sense to be made out of that bombing. I don't think we learned anything, do you?

It probably made me a little more cautious, because one thing that happened in that bombing that upset me more than anything was that little guy, that little guard out in front. A very nice looking young man. He was very friendly. He didn't speak much English, but he always said, "Hello, how are you?" and "You very pretty." Just rudimentary things like that, but he wasn't flirtatious. He was just sweet and nice and always talked to me. He was the lookout man! That really bothered me when I found it out, because I realized he didn't care about me. He didn't care about anybody. He was there on a mission. I just thought, I will never understand obviously these people in this part of the world, because I'm too trusting, I guess. I realized that I had been totally naive. I did find that at first I didn't cry. I would talk about it. I was very matter-of-fact. People would ask me about it and I would tell them what happened. But as time went on, in fact when the five-year mark came when we were in China, I was having dinner with two female friends one night. Jackie said something about what happened five years ago this week and I said what? She said "My God, you were there. The Beirut blow-up." I hadn't realized that it had been five years. I started crying, and I cried and I cried and I cried and I cried. Even now, when I talk to people now, I feel tears whereas I didn't the first couple of years after it happened. I guess I was just in denial or blocking it out. Because I see certain pictures in my mind when I think about it now. One of those is standing at the airport watching the coffins being loaded on board. That was hard. I don't think about the bombing much. But I think about it every April. Sometimes I don't understand why I'm thinking about Beirut, and then I'll realize it's about that time of year. I feel it was wasted effort. I don't think it accomplished anything for the people who did it. I don't think we learned much from it, because we put people back in there and it happened a second time.

The thing that has bothered me is that nobody seems to remember that we were bombed first. I mean, there's been no publicity. You never see that date mentioned. I mean, this year nobody mentioned it. The date that everyone talks about is the day the Marines were bombed. I understand that 200 and something young men lost their lives, but nobody seems to understand that what happened to us was a milestone in history because it had never happened before. It was a total violation of all diplomatic [?] and the Geneva Convention and everything else, yet nobody seems to remember that it happened. Somewhere along the line, somebody who knew I was in the Beirut bombing said, "Oh, that was after those Marines were killed." I said "No, that was before!"

There <u>was</u> another one after, but no one seems to remember that we were the first ones. There hasn't been much written about it at all.

I guess the one way it affected me is that I had wished that I had stayed in touch with people who were there and I haven't. They never did have a gathering of people. I don't know if they felt that most people just wanted to get on with their lives and forget it, or what. But I think it would have been good for people to get together. I would like to see how people are. People we never saw again.

I never thought about something like that happening to me. I hadn't even considered it, but I did find that I was much stronger than I ever would have thought. Going to work the next morning, pitching in, helping set up offices, and going to see the families of the people who died—I just automatically did these things because I knew they had to be done. I never would have thought that I would be strong enough to do that.

I do think that none of us had had any preparation for something like that. I know I had not. The only thing that USIS tried to get you to do was to take defensive driving, which was ridiculous. First of all, you couldn't have a car in Beirut. It would have been ridiculous anyway because all they had to do was shoot you. But I don't think that there was any preparation for the psychological effect of being without your spouse or living for months on end in a hotel. I think there should be more for the spouses. Our desk officer was fabulous about calling my husband and my parents. But nobody really reached out to the families who were back in the States [who] did not know what was going on in Beirut. I don't think we had any preparations at all. I think there should be more preparation for people to get them to face the fact that this could happen. These are the things that you must face. Are you ready for it? You and your family should have preparations for it in case your spouse is killed and you're not there. It's not things people want to talk about, but I think they should be forced to if they are going to go into situations like that.

We were bombed, I think, just because of the general vitriolic minds of those Islamic fanatics in Iran that hated the U.S. so much. They wanted to do something dreadful to show that we were not all-powerful and that we could be injured. Which is kind of strange, because they had already shown that when they took the hostages in Iran and we were not able to get them. I think it was just the general hatred of the people that did it for the U.S.

Edited interview   Kurt Shafer
November 27, 1993   AID Program Officer in 1983

Really and truly. You and Bob were sitting drinking coffee, having a little tête-à-tête. I stopped by and was thinking about having a cup of coffee, because we had French in the afternoon and I wanted to be a little more alert for the French lesson. But you guys were very, very serious and so I went on up to the office. About ten minutes after I had come back from the cafeteria, I put some M&Ms out on the table as a little dessert and there was sort of a low—I shouldn't say low, it was a deep strong blast—a low rumbling sound that grew in intensity. It lasted four to six seconds. I was on the floor under the desk with M&Ms scattered all over, waiting for the second blast. Smart bombers always had a little back-up explosive. I knew it was a bomb. I thought it wise to keep my head down for another 30 seconds and see if there was a second bomb. I don't know how long I waited, but it sort of spooked me. Finally, maybe after a minute or half minute, I came out. Of course glass was broken, M&Ms were every place and Yolanda, our secretary, came in and ran out and came back in and ran back out of the office again. Anyway, I was by myself and went to the door that separated my office from Tish's. The doors wouldn't open because the walls were buckled. But I got mad at Tish and said, "God damn it, she locked that door." I went on down the hallway to the main office area where everybody was. Some people were around Mrs. McIntyre who was bloody and walking around. Her eye was hemorrhaging. I didn't stay there long.

I went down to the Consular Section to look for Yolla Al'Hashim that I had been going out with for some period of time. I was on the fourth floor, and I walked down to the ground floor and tried to walk across what would have been the entrance to the Consular Section. The tear gas we had stored in the Embassy had blown, and it was really, really dense. I couldn't make it. So I went back. I don't know really whether I went back for a minute, or whether I went back and sat down. But I tried a second time, and again the tear gas was too strong, so I went back. I don't know how long I waited before I went back a third time. I don't know if there was a breeze blowing in from the Mediterranean or what, but it more or less cleared out. I got to the door of the Consular Section, and it was just one big massive pile of rubble. I turned around and started thinking about getting out of there. I was in sort of a state of shock and I don't really remember feeling anything, fear or anything. Just sort of a confusion, I'd say.

About that time, Dick Gannon was leading a half dozen other people trying to get them out. They were off on one side with a flashlight looking for a way out. I was some distance from them, but I did see light and dust and I went off in that direction. There was a hole in the back of the building and we went there and got out. I was the second or third person out. It was quite a long drop. We were helping three people come down. Out of the clear blue sky came the Lebanese "Rescue Committee." Literally, they almost physically pushed me away and took over doing the job themselves.

I meandered out in front of the building and talked to some people from the press and was quoted in a number of newspapers across the States. People sent copies of the newspaper article with my little quote in it to Mom. I said something to the effect that there wasn't anything anybody could do. The place wasn't defended. It wasn't barricaded, and there just wasn't anything anybody could do to stop it physically at the time it happened.

Then I went out along near the boardwalk and headed back to my apartment house. I was just a little ways, and who was there but a couple of friends and Annalisa Meyer, the German lady who lived in my apartment house. I told them what I knew and went back to the apartment and called my parents. They were watching it all on T.V. and quite obviously relieved to hear that I was fine.

Loud noises in Beirut sort of bothered one, but it was more from the bombing all of the time rather than from that one incident. If there were a loud explosion or loud bang, a firecracker, a car backfiring, it seemed like I jumped a little higher than usual. That lasted a few years, but I haven't jumped in a few years. Loud noises really did use to scare the daylights out of me. They had some psychiatrist out there, and I thought that was pretty silly and a waste of time. I guess if I had gotten hit in the head or knew the people who died really well—other than Bill McIntyre and Yolla I didn't know them—I mean, I would think a car wreck could have been a heck of a lot worse. Some people were cut a little bit here, a little bit there, but the actual incident was over in five seconds, outside, of course, those who were injured. Then it was just sort of the aftermath. I've often wondered why it left me in that state of shock. Why I sort of felt confused for about half an hour. It wasn't, I say, the incident itself, it was just realizing what happened and knowing that people were hurt. It sort of built up. I reckon it's the single most trying experience I've had, but it was not all that traumatic, all that life-threatening. More in the mind. A natural threat of damage to the person.

I do remember thinking, my God, every week, or at least it seemed like every week, something worse happened. Either the shelling, the Israeli invasion, the assassination of Malcolm Kerr, the President of AUB. We were blown up and Marines were getting blown up. It was one thing after another. One must remember that there were a series of things in Beirut, and really and truly the shelling sometimes was a lot more frightening than the actual incident at the Embassy was. So, no, I enjoyed Beirut very much that summer.

That summer in Beirut, spring of 1983, was one of the neatest summers I had ever spent. Just to put it very bluntly, here you had beautiful Arab girls who were not covered behind a veil and available at various saltwater swimming pools at all those hotels. I couldn't wait for Saturday and Sunday to go up to the St. George Hotel and lay around there and drink beer and eat food and meet somebody different. I enjoyed that summer very, very immensely.

I've seem some Lebanese in Paris a couple of times in the last ten years and was treated even closer than an uncle, like a brother who had been gone for a couple of years. They just couldn't be more decent.

Then we all were evacuated again, I think in October or maybe in September of 1983. We were in Cyprus for a month exactly. After the Marine barracks were blown up, only Lee Twentymen and I went back. I was out checking with UNICEF, the U.N. office not far from AUB, when shelling started. It was the time when the Shiites tried to take over East Beirut. I was in the U.N. building at the time and the Lebanese, of course, were listening to the radios. It broadcasted we were under an immediate curfew. Of course, this was done by the central government. The fighting was going on and just twenty minutes after that, you looked out the window and here were the Shiites in their uniforms, which consisted of white sneakers, blue jeans and some sort of jacket, with Kalashnikovs on their backs. I mean, they had literally taken over West Beirut. So there I stayed and finally realized that I was probably going to be evacuated with the U.N. There was some talk about letting me use one of the official U.N. cars to get back up to where the [American] Embassy was or at least [to] the British Embassy...but that wasn't deemed wise. I spent the night there and the next morning, I think it was around 11:00 the next morning, some shops opened. Some people were out doing shopping. One of the heads of the various missions offered me a chauffeur to walk me up to the AUB gate so that I could make it back to where the British Embassy was. Because I was with a Lebanese, nobody bothered me. I remember going to that goddamned gate, and of course, my escort was nervous. There were a couple of Shiite guards standing in front of the gate hassling somebody else off to the side. I didn't say, "*Sabaah ilheer*" (good morning). I just walked on by, got inside AUB, and said goodbye to my escort. I started walking fast right straight through there and was amazed how the Palestinians had dug that place up for defensive against the big Israeli invasion. I walked on through, not seeing anybody. It was really uneventful. It must have been approaching noon and the first person I saw was Bob Pugh. He said something like, "Thank God," and I guessed that I was perhaps the last person unaccounted for. Back up to our offices was Lee Twentymen. He was very upset. He was sort of half-pissed because I disobeyed orders. He had said to take a car, not to walk. But this U.N. office was so close I could just walk up the back steps to the old Embassy. I didn't take a car. We left that afternoon by helicopter to the ship.

If I were in another embassy that blew up, I would do just exactly what was done in Beirut: take care of physical needs and then spiritual needs, if you will. After Beirut I was in Chad and then Uganda. Uganda was hot as hell that first year I was there. I didn't go out anyplace at night without severe threat of having a car hijacked from underneath me, and coming back at night, if you saw car lights in your rearview mirror, you drove 40-50 miles an hour over the most pot-hole roads you could imagine, heading for home or an American's house, get inside behind a gate, behind a fence and a guard. There was no special preparation. I don't know of special lectures about going to places like Chad.

I told the security officer, at a Friday night Marine party get-together, I'd say about three weeks before it happened, a Palestinian with no legs and no balls and not very rich would gladly give up his life as long as his family was assured of being taken care of at the expense of the PLO or whoever, and there was just no protection at the Embassy for anybody, no walls, no fences, anybody could drive right up there with whatever they had. And that's what happened.

[Shortly after the interview, Shafer phoned to say that he had attended the funeral of Yolla Al'Hashim and that it was one of the most difficult things he had ever done.]

Edited interview	Rebecca (Rikkie) Smith
January 5, 1994	Secretary to USAID Director in 1983

Malcolm called in October of 1982 and asked if I could be in Beirut by November of 1982. The war in Lebanon became much closer to me then the one in Vietnam.

On April 18, I was at my desk and the window behind me blew in behind me. That's how my forehead got cut. Something hit me on the back of my head. It must have hit me, to knock off the glasses, or maybe it was just the impact from the bomb. My barrette flew off and my hair sort of stood up like I was startled. I heard the noise, that sort of impact noise. I thought it was a sonic boom, because earlier in the day the jets had been flying over doing some kind of testing run. Wasn't it a wet, overcast day? That makes a sonic boom closer. Then I saw all that glass from the window. Sylvia, the secretary, was screaming. She didn't seem to be hurt, but I think she was looking at me. I must have been more bloody then I thought.

I became very clearheaded and thought I must be helpful. I must not panic. I must not act scared. I must not throw up. Think: I did escape. Realize you were hurt but just slightly. Then you say, what should I do first? Should I run down and give blood?

I immediately knew it was a bomb, but then you get scared and that's why you try to get out really fast, because maybe there will be a second one, but then when I thought about the classified [material] I thought, no, I'm not going to have somebody that I don't want to come find that stuff. Not that it was really secretive. It wasn't really nation-shattering. I went back to my office and found my glasses, my barrette, and I put the classified in the safe. Later when we went back, the papers were all bloody and stuck together because I had bled on them. I slammed the safe shut. I went out without my coat. Days later I was fretting about that coat and that sandwich the guy from the cafeteria had just delivered.

I was frightened and shocked, but I also realized I could walk so I should probably go help people. I wondered if I should go looking about, but then I realized that places were sort of hanging loose and I had better not. For a while we leaned up against the wall, and then we sat down on the floor because we couldn't figure out a way to get out. So we thought we would wait until someone comes along who looks authoritative, like a Marine guard or a security officer. It must have been thirty minutes. We had tried to get out but the steps had disappeared. A Marine guard came and took us one flight down and we walked on the top of some kind of garage where there was a ladder. We were on the roof. I had a gash here on my thumb. It was sitting up like a burst hot dog that you cook too much, but I thought, it's not bad. I can still navigate.

When I came down the ladder, Abed the driver put me in an ambulance, and I kept saying, "No! No! No ambulance for me, I can walk. Save it for somebody who is really on a stretcher." He insisted and rode with me, and the ambulance ride was horrible. It was going tickie, tickie, and swerving around. I thought, this is so silly. Even when I got to the hospital, I thought they would say, "Oh, you're not hurt. Stand up. Get up." They didn't. An intern came in and he told me his life. He was going to Texas the next week, if he could get out. Everybody thought that the planes would be stopped immediately. He stitched my thumb right up. He put five stitches in there. Put it right back very neat. See, the scar is almost gone. I know there is still some glass in there, because on wet days I can feel like a little "ting," little prickly thing. They had me down flat, too, but I realized I could walk.

For some reason, when I went home that night from the hospital, we went to Tish's apartment for a few minutes and talked. I felt like I had to sleep. Everybody on the AID staff, except me, went back to work the next day. I wanted to sleep the next day for some reason. I said, "I'll take a day off to think about the bombing." I wanted to relive things to see what I could remember, because you do block out a lot of things immediately.

The next day everything seemed so precious, every little thing was so particularly special that you noticed it. You don't take anything for granted for a long time, and then you start flipping back into your old ways.

I can't remember having any reactions, like I was really scared. But from then on we were told to check under our cars to see if anybody placed a bomb under it. I thought, if I get down on the ground and slide under and look and see a bomb, I would be so frightened that I would rather take my chances and turn the ignition key and see if I go sky high. If it did, I wouldn't know about it until later.

The DCM kept calling us all together. We had a daily meeting about what we were going to do that day, what we should do and what ceremonies and who was being shipped out. They had some kind of ceremony a few days later at the airport when they shipped the caskets out.

McFarland from the NSC and Shultz talked to us. Actually, it's hard to find the words to say to make people feel better. What do you do? Right away you say, well, I have to get back to work. I thought you should think about it a lot. Just talk about it, because I think that it is a great relief to talk about it. There were lots of people who wanted to talk about it. All the communication people were very helpful. They were outstanding.

I don't want to go to any more war zones or any more places where they are mad at you. Of course, it is hard to find a place where they are not mad at you for their own reasons. But I always volunteered for things before, thinking it was very adventuresome. But it is really frightening. When we heard loud noises, we were just a nervous wreck.

People would jump so far at cars backfiring. I thought it was a good idea that they were going to ship people home for a little rest to think about things. The scary part was going back to Beirut, because you really knew that the ones who blew up the Embassy still had some of their comrades who wanted to blow us up.

I was having nightmares. I'm a nightmare person. I have horrible dreams every night. I have such dreams that I wonder where they are coming from, but I mean, to this day I have horrible dreams, but I don't relive the bombing anymore. I've gotten that out of my mind somehow. I thought I would be reliving it for a year, but I wasn't. I would say in four to six months it was gone. Almost the memory of it was gone. I think also that it causes you to feel aches and pains or something. I think that you kind of feel sorry for yourself that you let yourself get in that position.

A psychiatrist came from Egypt to talk to us about three days later. She was terrific. She made us all talk about our feelings and fears and our wants and our needs. There were mainly women there. Maybe one man came, Bob Essington. The psychiatrist wanted us to talk a lot about the bombing in case we still had something we were blocking up inside.

The bombing has made me more cautious. I don't go in harm's way as much. I don't accept assignments to war-torn countries. I don't defy the odds anymore, but I never was what you would call a gambler, so I guess I've always been cautious. I wouldn't say that it changed my life in any grave way.

Mine was the first R&R and it was on May 9th. I stayed one week back here in the States. All the family was eager for details because they had been hearing little reports. First they were told that I was injured but not much. The next day they heard that the bandages were coming off and the splints and the stitches were coming out. My family said, "What bandages? What splints? You said she was fine!" Then they wanted to hear every little detail. To me, that was good therapy to talk about every little thing, because then you're reliving it that final time. They were curious. It was nice to have curiosity. It was good, that feeling. While you were travelling, if you were to say that you were out in Beirut, people would say, "Beirut! Were you in Beirut?" Then they would want to know the details, too. A lot of people talked to you just sort of out of the blue. You were a celebrity for a while.

I think that really we are naive and trusting and we don't think that anyone is out to blow us up. I remember thinking when I could hear the whistle of incoming fire, that time we had constant artillery barrage, rocket-propelled grenades over my house, "What do they want? What do they want? Give them what they want." I just felt so sad about bombs and all that situation, because I knew that somewhere there could have been talks but now it was too late. Now you had to wait for talks. I didn't know how to stop it.

There was a Marine that I really liked. He was my favorite. A marine named Bob McMaugh. He had been teasing me just days before about the Super Bowl. All the Marines were a great bunch. They all knew that they were lucky to be alive. I always thought that they were so good that nobody would ever break into our building, and here they came in so easily. But every time I arrived in a taxi at the

Embassy, I thought of how vulnerable we were. Look, you drove right in this alley. We didn't even stop coming in the driveway. To me that was too trusting. The building was unsecured. Our offices were right on the street. They let them come right in without saying, "Halt, let's see your credentials."

We got together at houses a lot, and I remember inviting a lot of Marines out for lunch, like everyday ,because I wanted to say, I'm glad you're alive and I'm sorry about Bob [McMaugh].

You know the other end of our floor was political. That political part [CIA] got hurt, which made a lot of people believe that maybe they were the actual target, because there was a bunch of bigwig visitors that weekend.

Years before I had something called "evasive" training. It was like counter- terrorism training. They taught us how to evade if someone was trying to push us off the road. I feel that if they are really aiming to get you, well, it's too easy. Look how they blew up the Marine barracks.

Endnotes

1. A.N. Alexander, "A Personal Account of the Bombing of the American Embassy in Beirut," *Business America*, 30 May 1983, 16-18.
2. Philo Dibble, "Beirut Bombing: Report from Embassy Says 7 Floors Collapsed One After the Other," *State*, May 1983, 2-9.
3. tephen E. Auldridge, "Brothers in Beirut," *State*, June 1983, 1.
4. U.S. Congress, House of Representatives, Committee on Foreign Affairs, "The U.S. Embassy Bombing in Beirut," 98th Cong., 1st Sess., 28 June, 1983, 4.
5. Charles D. Smith, *Palestine and the Arab-Israeli Conflict* (San Diego State University: St. Martin's Press, 1992), 267.
6. *Ibid.*
7. John L. Esposito, *Islam and Politics* (Syracuse: Syracuse University Press, 1984), 248.
8. *Ibid.*, 249.
9. Robert Fisk, *Pity the Nation* (Oxford: Oxford University Press, 1990), 480.
10. Charles Simpkinson and Anne Simpkinson, eds., *Sacred Stories: A Celebration of the Power of Story to Transform and Heal* (San Francisco: Harper, 1993), 155.
11. Philip Habib was President Reagan's Special Envoy to Lebanon.
12. I had intended to talk to all those on temporary duty with the three agencies but could not locate them.

13. Stephen M. Sonnenberg, Arthur S. Blank and John A. Talbott, eds., *The Trauma of War: Stress and Recovery in Viet Nam Veterans* (Washington, D.C.: American Psychiatric Press, Inc., 1985), 6.
14. Shirley Dicks, *From Vietnam to Hell: Interviews with Victims of Post-Traumatic Stress Disorder* (Jefferson, North Carolina: McFarland and Company, Inc., Publishers, 1990), 3.
15. Ghislaine Boulanger, "Post-Traumatic Stress Disorder: An Old Problem with a New Name," Sonnenberg et al., 20.
16. Arthur L. Arnold, "Diagnosis of Post-Traumatic Stress Disorder in Viet Nam Veterans," Sonnenberg et al., 105.
17. Boulanger, 16.
18. *Diagnostic and Statistical Manual of Mental Disorders (DSM-III-R)*, 3rd ed., revised (Washington, D.C.: American Psychiatric Association, 1987), 249.
19. Carol S. North, Elizabeth M. Smith and Edward L. Spitznagel, "Posttraumatic Stress Disorder in Survivors of a Mass Shooting," *American Journal of Psychiatry*, January 1994, 87.
20. *DSM-III-R*, 247-251.
21. *Ibid.*, 247.
22. Jeffrey Mitchell, "Healing the Helper," *Role Stressors and Supports for Emergency Workers* (Rockville: National Institute of Mental Health, 1984), 106.
23. Robyn C. Robinson and Jeffrey T. Mitchell, "Evaluation of Psychological Debriefings," *Journal of Traumatic Stress*, 6:3, 1993, 368.
24. Jeffrey T. Mitchell and George S. Everly, *Critical Incident Stress Debriefing (CISD): An Operation Manual for the Prevention of Traumatic Stress Among Emergency Services*

and Disaster Workers (Ellicott City: Chevron Publishing Corporation, 1993), 14.

25. *Ibid.*, 3.
26. *Ibid.*, 34.
27. *Ibid.*, 15.
28. Marilyn Holmes, interview by author, 11 March 1994, Washington, D.C.
29. Robinson and Mitchell, 367.
30. Actually, Toot says, "I think I can. I think I can."
31. *Allah Akbar* means "God is great," and is often shouted by Muslims as they enter battle.
32. Post One, located just inside the entrance of the Embassy, was where Marine guards were stationed.
33. Sabra and Shatila are Palestinian camps in West Beirut. During the Israeli occupation, many hundreds of Palestinians (as well as poor Lebanese and foreigners) were massacred by the Christian Phalange from the evening of September 15 to the morning of September 18, 1982.
34. Sheila Platt, a clinical social worker, does critical incident stress debriefings for the United Nations. She has lectured and made several training videos on stress management for the State Department.
35. Marilyn Holmes, writer and producer, works for Diplomatic Security in the State Department. She was responsible for several training videos on the effects of trauma on the lives of individuals.
36. The two psychiatrists sent to Beirut were Paul F. Eggertsen and Christine Bieniek.
37. State Department psychiatrist, Christine Bieniek, interviewed by author, 9 August

1994, Washington, D.C., State Department, Washington, D.C.

38. U.S. Department of State, "Report of the Secretary of State's Advisory Panel on Overseas Security," (Washington, D.C.: United States Department of State, 1985).

39. *Ibid.*, 4.

40. *Ibid.*, 34-36.

41. Coordinator of SOS, DanaDee Carragher, interview by author, 10 August 1994, Arlington, Virginia.

42. SOS lecturer, Cay Hartley, interview by author, 27 July 1994, Washington, D.C.

43. Jean Fran Webb, ed. "Culture Shock," *Foreign Service Assignment Notebook* (Washington, D.C.: Foreign Service Institute, 1993), 76-77.

44. Director of Overseas Briefing Center, Ray Leki, interview by author, 10 August 1994, Arlington, Virginia.

45. Associate Medical Director of Mental Health Services, Esther P. Roberts, interview by author, 9 August 1994, Washington, D.C.

46. Clinical Social Worker, Sheila Platt, interview by author by phone, 1 March 1994, New York, tape recording.

47. Taken from the June 1983 Department of State newsletter, State.

48. The corniche is the main avenue which runs along the Mediterranean Sea.

49. A plastic material designed to prevent glass from turning into shards in an explosion.

50. Ain Helway is a Palestinian camp in southern Lebanon which was leveled by the Israelis in 1982.

51. Rafiq Hariri, a Lebanese entrepreneur with close ties to the Saudi royal family, led in the reconstruction of Beirut. He is presently the Prime Minister of Lebanon.

52. The Inman Commission was an Advisory Panel on Overseas Security which submitted a report to the Secretary of State in June 1985.

BIBLIOGRAPHY

Alexander, A.N. "A Personal Account of the Bombing of the American Embassy in Beirut." *Business America* 6 (May 30, 1983), 16-18.

Arnold, Arthur L. "Diagnosis of Post-Traumatic Stress Disorder in Viet Nam Veterans." In *The Trauma of War: Stress and Recovery in Viet Nam Veterans*, ed. Stephen M. Sonnenberg, Arthur S. Blank and John A. Talbott, 99-124. Washington, D.C.: American Psychiatric Press, Inc., 1985.

Auldridge, Stephen E. "Brothers in Beirut," *State* (June 1983), 1, 57.

Bieniek, Christine, State Department Psychiatrist. Interview by author, 9 August 1984, Washington, D.C.

Boulanger, Ghislaine. "Post-Traumatic Stress Disorder: An Old Problem with a New Name." In *The Trauma of War: Stress and Recovery in Viet Nam Veterans*, ed. Stephen M. Sonnenberg, Arthur S. Blank and John A. Talbott, 13-30. Washington, D.C.: American Psychiatric Press, Inc., 1985.

Butler, Tish. Interview by author, 14 February 1994, Washington, D.C. Tape recording.

Carragher, DanaDee, Coordinator of SOS. Interview by author, 10 August 1994, Arlington, Virginia.

Chesler, Phyllis. *Trauma and Recovery*. New York: Harper Collins Publishers, Inc., 1993.

Colodzin, Benjamin. *How to Survive Trauma*. Station Hill, New York: Station Hill Press, 1993.

Crocker, Christine. Interview by author, 5 January 1994, Arlington. Tape recording.

Crocker, Ryan. Interview by author, 4 January 1994, Washington, D.C. Tape recording.

Diagnostic and Statistical Manual of Mental Disorders, 3rd
 ed., revised. "Post-Traumatic Stress Disorder," 247-51.

Dibble, Philo. "Beirut Bombing: Report From Embassy Says 7 Floors Collapsed One After the Other." *State* (May 1983), 2-9.

Dicks, Shirley. *From Vietnam to Hell: Interviews with
 Victims of Post-Traumatic Stress Disorder*. Jefferson, North Carolina: McFarland and Company, Inc., 1990.

Dillard, Diane. Interview by author, 14 February 1994, Washington, D.C. Tape recording.

Dillon, Robert. Interview by author, 19 January 1994, Washington, D.C. Tape recording.

Esposito, John L. *Islam and Politics*. Syracuse: Syracuse University Press, 1984.

Figley, Charles R. *Helping Traumatized Families*. San Francisco: Jossey-
 Bass Publishers, 1989.

----------------. *Trauma and Its Wake*. New York: Brunner/ Mazel,
 Publishers, 1985.

Fisk, Robert. *Pity the Nation*. Oxford: Oxford University Press, 1991.

Gannon, Richard. Interview by author, 11 January 1994, Washington, D.C. Tape recording.

Gregory, Barbara. Interview by phone by author, 12 February 1994, Mount Dora, Florida.

Tape

recording.

Hammel, Eric. *The Root: The Marines in Beirut, August 1982-February 1984*. Orlando,
 Florida: Harcourt Brace Jovanovich, Publishers, 1985.

Hartley, Cay, SOS lecturer. Interview by author, 27 July 1994, Washington, D.C.

Holmes, Marilyn, Producer-Writer. Interview by author, 11 March 1994, Washington, D.C. Lee, Faith. Interview by phone by author, 16 January 1994, Chicago.

Leki, Ray, Director of Overseas Briefing Center. Interview by author, 10 August 1994, Arlington.

Lira, Elizabeth, David Becker, and Maria Isabel Castillo.
"Psychotherapy with Victims of Political Repression in Chile: A Therapeutic and Political Challenge." In *Health Services for the Treatment of Torture and Trauma Survivors*, ed. Janet Gruschow and Kari Hannibal, 108-111. Washington, D.C.: American Association for the Advancement of Science, 1990.

Mandel, David. Interview by phone by author, 17 November 1993, Washington, D.C. Tape recording.

McCann, I. Lisa and Laurie Anne Pearlman. *Psychological Trauma and the Adult Survivor.* New York: Brunner/ Mazel, Publishers, 1990.

Mitchell, Jeffrey. "Healing the Helper." In *Role Stressors and Supports for Emergency Workers*, 105-118. Rockville: National Institute of Mental Health, 1984.

Mitchell, Jeffrey T. and George S. Everly. *Critical Incident Stress Debriefing (CISD): An Operation Manual for the Prevention of Traumatic Stress Among Emergency Services and Disaster Workers.* Ellicott City: Chevron Publishing Corp., 1993.

North, Carol S., Elizabeth M. Smith and Edward L. Spitznagel.
"Posttraumatic Stress Disorder in Survivors of a Mass Shooting," *American Journal of Psychiatry* 151 (January 1994), 82-88.

Pascoe, Dorothy. Interview by phone by author, 11 December 1993, Henderson, Nevada.

Tape recording.

Pech, Dorothy. Interview by author, 11 January 1994, Washington, D.C. Tape recording.

Pellegrino, Daniel J. Interview by author, 14 January 1994, Albany. Tape recording.

Platt, Sheila, Clinical Social Worker. Interview by phone by author, 1 March 1994, New York. Tape recording.

Roberts, Esther P., Associate Medical Director of Mental Health Services. Interview by author, 9 August 1994, Washington, D.C.

Robinson, Robyn C. and Jeffrey T. Mitchell. "Evaluation of Psychological Debriefings." *Journal of Traumatic Stress* 6:3, (July 1993), 367-82.

Roth, S. and Cohen, L.J. "Approach, Avoidance and Coping with Stress." *American Psychologist* 41 (July 1986), 813-819.

Samuel, Beth. Interview by author, 12 February 1994, Corpus Christi. Tape recording. Simpkinson, Charles and Anne Simpkinson, eds. *Sacred Stories:*

A Celebration of the Power of Story to Transform and Heal. San Francisco: Harper, 1993.

Shafer, Kurt. Interview by author, 27 November 27, 1993, Chatsworth, Illinois. Tape recording.

Smith, Charles D. *Palestine and the Arab-Israeli Conflict.*

San Diego State University: St. Martin's Press, 1992.

Smith, Rebecca. Interview by author, 5 January 1994. Tape recording.

Sonnenberg, Stephen M., Arthur S. Blank and John A. Talbott, eds. *The Trauma of War: Stress and Recovery in Viet Nam Veterans.* Washington, D.C.: American Psychiatric Press, Inc., 1985.

U.S. Congress. House. Committee on Appropriations, Subcommittee on Department of Defense. "Situation in Lebanon and Grenada." 98th Cong., 1st Sess., 8 November 1983, 24-29.

U.S. Congress. House. Committee on Armed Services and Committee on Veterans Affairs. "Beirut Tragedy: 'A New Crowd in Town' and Beirut Casualties: Care and Identification." 98th Cong., 1st Sess., 1983.

U.S. Congress. House. Committee on Foreign Affairs. "The U.S. Embassy Bombing in Beirut." 98th Cong., 1st Sess., 28 June 1983, 1-24.

U.S. Department of State. "Report of the Secretary of State's Advisory Panel on Overseas Security." Washington, D.C.: Department of State, 1985.

Webb, Jean Fran. *Foreign Service Assignment Notebook*. Washington, D.C: Foreign Service Institute, 1993.

Weir, Benjamin M. "Reflections of a Former Hostage on Causes of Terrorism," *Arab Studies Quarterly*, 9:2 (Spring 1987), 155-61.

www.ingramcontent.com/pod-product-compliance
Lightning Source LLC
Chambersburg PA
CBHW020541030426
42337CB00013B/935